Standing Ovation

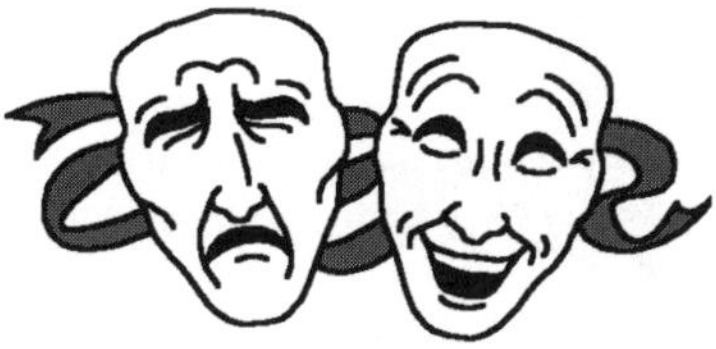

ETHNOGRAPHIC ALTERNATIVES BOOK SERIES

Series Editors
Carolyn Ellis
Arthur P. Bochner
(both at the University of South Florida)

About the Series:

Ethnographic Alternatives emphasizes experimental forms of qualitative writing that blur the boundaries between social sciences and humanities. The editors encourage submissions that experiment with novel forms of expressing lived experience, including literary, poetic, autobiographical, multivoiced, conversational, critical, visual, performative, and co-constructed representations. Emphasis should be on expressing concrete lived experience through narrative modes of writing.

We are interested in ethnographic alternatives that promote narration of local stories; literary modes of descriptive scene setting, dialogue, and unfolding action; and inclusion of the author's subjective reactions, involvement in the research process, and strategies for practicing reflexive fieldwork.

Please send proposals to:
Carolyn Ellis and Arthur P. Bochner
College of Arts and Sciences
Department of Communication
University of South Florida
4202 East Fowler Avenue, CIS 1040
Tampa, FL 33620-7800
Email: cellis@chuma.cas.usf.edu

Books in the Series:

Volume 1, *Composing Ethnography: Alternative Forms of Qualitative Writing*, Carolyn Ellis and Arthur P. Bochner, editors
Volume 2, *Opportunity House: Ethnographic Stories of Mental Retardation*, Michael V. Angrosino
Volume 3, *Kaleidoscope Notes: Writing Women's Music and Organizational Culture*, Stacy Holman Jones
Volume 4, *Fiction and Social Research: By Fire or Ice*, Anna Banks and Stephen P. Banks, editors
Volume 5, *Reading Auschwitz*, Mary Lagerwey
Volume 6, *Life Online: Researching Real Experience in Virtual Space*, Annette N. Markham
Volume 7, *Writing the New Ethnography*, H. L. Goodall, Jr.
Volume 8, *Between Gay and Straight: Understanding Friendship Beyond Sexual Orientation*, Lisa Tillmann-Healy
Volume 9, *Ethnographically Speaking: Autoethnography, Literature, and Aesthetics*, Arthur P. Bochner and Carolyn Ellis, editors
Volume 10, *Karaoke Nights: An Ethnographic Rhapsody*, Rob Drew
Volume 11, *Standing Ovation: Performing Social Science Research about Cancer*, Ross Gray and Christina Sinding

Standing Ovation

Performing Social Science Research about Cancer

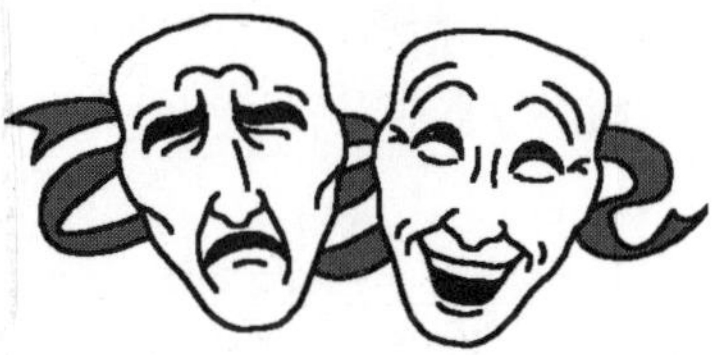

Ross Gray
Christina Sinding

ALTAMIRA PRESS

A Division of Rowman & Littlefield Publishers, Inc.
Walnut Creek • Lanham • New York • Oxford

AltaMira Press
A Division of Rowman & Littlefield Publishers, Inc.
1630 North Main Street, #367
Walnut Creek, CA 94596
www.altamirapress.com

Rowman & Littlefield Publishers, Inc.
4720 Boston Way
Lanham, MD 20706

12 Hid's Copse Road
Cumnor Hill, Oxford OX2 9JJ, England

British Library Cataloguing in Publication Information Available

Library of Congress Cataloging-in-Publication Data

Gray, Ross, 1955–
Standing ovation : performing social science research about cancer / by Ross Gray and Christina Sinding.
p. cm. — (Ethnographic alternatives book series ; v. 11)
Includes bibliographical references and index.
ISBN 0-7591-0145-0 (cloth : alk. paper)—ISBN 0-7591-0146-9 (pbk. : alk. paper)
1. Breast—Cancer—Patients—Ontario—Toronto. 2. Breast—Cancer—Social aspects. 3. Breast—Cancer—Drama. 4. Theater—Ontario—Toronto. I. Sinding, Christina, 1967– II. Title. III. Series.

RC280.B8 G715 2002
362.1'9699449—dc21

2002001119

Printed in the United States of America

∞™ The paper used in this publication meets the minimum requirements of American National Standard for Information Sciences—Permanence of Paper for Printed Library Materials, ANSI/NISO Z39.48-1992.

CONTENTS

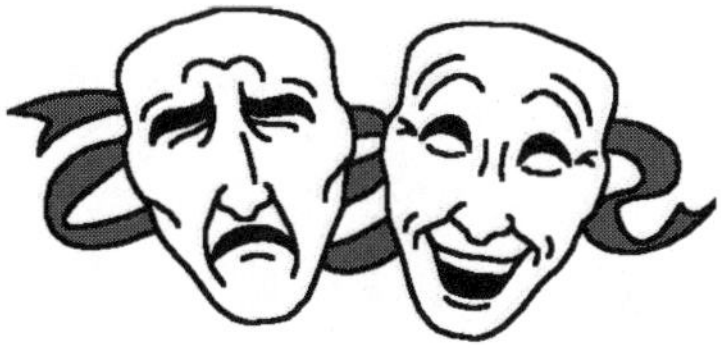

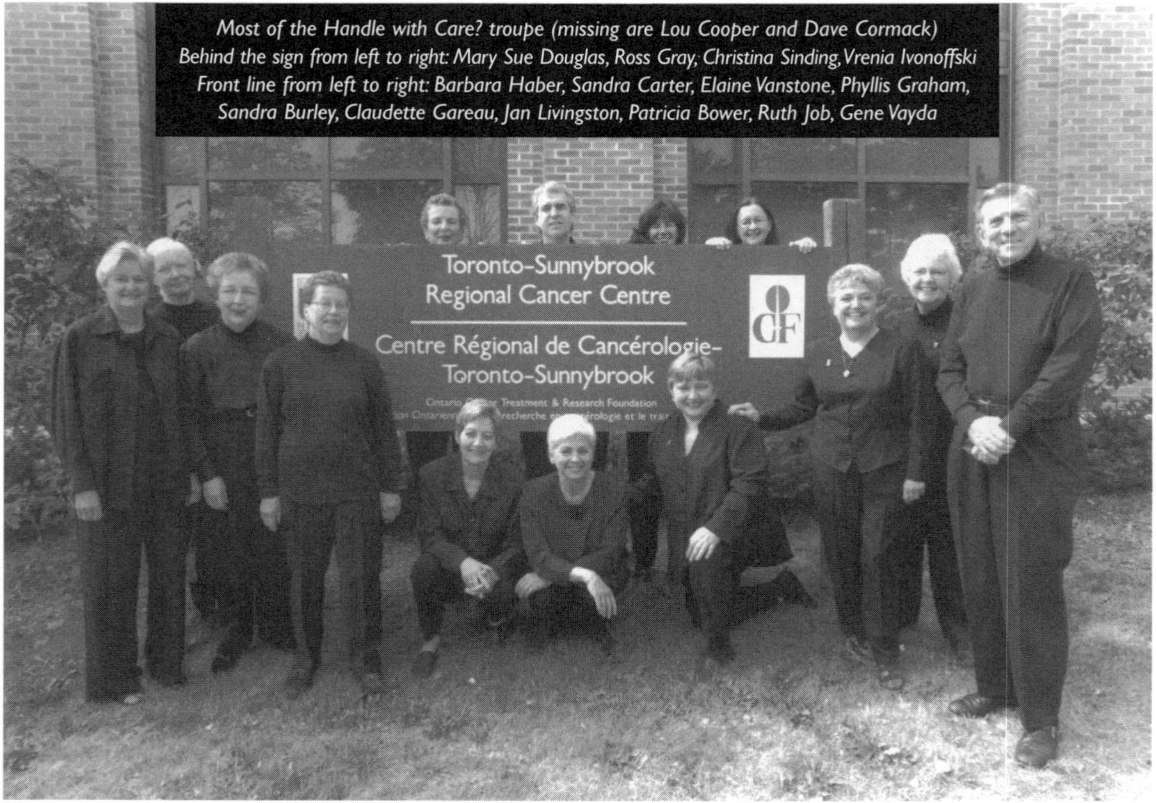

Most of the Handle with Care? troupe (missing are Lou Cooper and Dave Cormack)
Behind the sign from left to right: Mary Sue Douglas, Ross Gray, Christina Sinding, Vrenia Ivonoffski
Front line from left to right: Barbara Haber, Sandra Carter, Elaine Vanstone, Phyllis Graham, Sandra Burley, Claudette Gareau, Jan Livingston, Patricia Bower, Ruth Job, Gene Vayda

FOREWORD

I first saw *Handle with Care?* live at an academic conference in Florida organized by Art Bochner and Carolyn Ellis; several months later, I saw it again at the Tom Baker Cancer Centre in Calgary, Alberta, where, years before, I had been treated for cancer. Each performance was a different experience, and I'm sure that if I'd been at the second Tom Baker performance given for health professionals, that would have been different again. The differences, I think, had less to do with changes in the script—which scenes were included for different audiences—but were an effect of the play's particular genius for drawing upon the audience's energy. Our memories and fears infuse its words and actions; it speaks what we could not say.

To watch *Handle with Care?* is to cease to spectate and, very quickly, to become part of the play. Some audience members become the person with metastatic disease; others become family members, alternatively supportive and complaining; others are friends who do something helpful or blundering; and still others see themselves in the depictions of medical staff, primarily physicians. Especially when audience members are not sure which cast members have metastatic disease themselves, the tangle of projections and identifications becomes more intense. To watch the play is to be in the play. Everyone in the theater has cancer.

As family, friends, and physicians swirl around the person with cancer, we experience what these people look, sound, and even feel like to the ill person. To many who see the play, that vision of themselves is undoubtedly sobering. Yet *Handle with Care?* also has the grace—which some would call humor and others would call pacing—to make it tolerable to be the person with an ultimately terminal disease, and to be those around this person, doing too much or too little or, very occasionally, something just right.

Handle with Care? is not only a theatrical experience, it's also a research report, based on carefully conducted interviews and focus groups with women who have metastatic breast cancer. This research does what many social scientists talk about in principle but few are able to effect in practice: it listens. Feminist methodologies were perhaps the first to emphasize honoring the voices of respondents rather than treating them as "data," grist for the social science mill. This critique became personal for me after I had cancer and, in a still unstable remission, turned to reading psychologists who study and counsel people with cancer. What I read wasn't merely disturbing, it was maddening. What right, I asked—shouted—to myself, have these people to talk about me as some kind of specimen of behavioral disorders? What was so completely lacking in professional psychological writings about cancer—and in my own discipline of medical sociology—was any sense of what it is like to be a person living with cancer: what it's like to receive this news; to become progressively isolated from family, friends, and fellow workers who, even if well-intentioned, simply don't get it; what it's like to wake up every day with either the immediate prospect of some treatment that will make you feel even worse; or just knowing that more sickness and more treatments are on the horizon; what it's like to worry about leaving behind loved ones, especially children, far too soon.

Handle with Care? is a new kind of research report, but the voices remain those who are living with cancer. The point is not for some expert to show how much more he or she knows, but to allow people living with cancer to say what they have learned at such enormous cost. When I saw the play, I knew this was the research report I wanted those who might someday care for me to have seen, so that they could *care* for me, not just treat me.

I have been lucky never to reach the threshold that *Handle with Care?* crosses as it explores metastatic disease. I had secondary tumors, but they shrank on schedule with chemotherapy. I've had suspected recurrences, but I've never had to face the reality that cancer will keep coming back until it finally kills me. That's the place where *Handle with Care?* takes its audience. The place is scary, funny, terribly sad, and, ultimately, the play shows how it can be the only place worth being.

Ross and Chris deserve to brag at actually having pulled it off—creating *Handle with Care?* and then going on to create *No Big Deal?*—as does everyone else involved in the plays. Although *Standing Ovation* describes earlier work in research-based theater, nothing quite like these plays has been done before: nothing bringing together the research before production, the collaborative script writing, the cast mix of women with metastatic disease, health care professionals, and actors (some of whom had their own histories of cancer), the multiple versions for different audiences, and the extensive touring, and behind all these, the constant scramble for money and more money. Compared to most medical research, these plays are cheap. But Ross and Chris had to deal with funders who had no template to understand what they would be paying for.

Standing Ovation is less a how-to guide for other research-based theater than an inspiration for such work. Each project, the authors realize, must find its own way; there is no method. But here is a look backstage at the fears, frustrations, and, ultimately, the triumphs of production. And here is an enormous challenge to social science, especially to health psychology. Can you, Ross and Chris implicitly ask their professional colleagues, be so true to the lives and experiences of ill people? Can you let them speak and be so respectful to their speech? Can you take your part in the play of people's lives?

Much of the energy of *Handle with Care?* and much of the story told in *Standing Ovation* revolves around two women, Jan Livingston and Mary Sue Douglas, who lived with metastatic breast cancer while they performed in the play. At the performance in Florida, I saw both Jan and Mary Sue in the cast. By the time the play got to Calgary, Jan was too sick and Mary Sue performed while in treatment; I can only describe her as radiantly bald. Then Jan died, and as sad as that was, it wasn't as sad as it might have been because she *played* her part. Cancer leaves a person no choice but to have it until you might be lucky enough for it to go into remission. But Jan and Mary Sue found a space within which they could and did choose. Putting the audience in that space with them is how these plays infuse dying with such exuberant energy.

One of my favorite lines in *Standing Ovation* describes Jan creating a scene that shows her different fears and losses speaking to her through the voices of her fellow actors. Ross and Chris evoke what is therapeutic both about performing these plays and about participating as an audience member. "In performance," they write, Jan (who both has metastatic cancer and is playing a woman with this disease) "listens intently to [her fears and losses] for her own reasons rather than having them manifest without warning and against her will." Perhaps that describes how these plays about such a depressing subject can be such an uplifting experience to be part of. As audience members, we too see and hear our fears of suffering and loss, but the experience is the opposite of an uncontrollable nightmare. The play enables us to listen intently for our own reasons. Fears and losses will return, without warning and against our will; they will for most all of us someday, and I'm sure they did for Jan before she died. But for those who have been able to play those fears and losses, there is a difference. A difference for Jan, for me, and for all who experience these remarkable plays.

ARTHUR W. FRANK

Author of *At the Will of the Body* and
The Wounded Storyteller: Body, Illness, and Ethics

ACKNOWLEDGMENTS

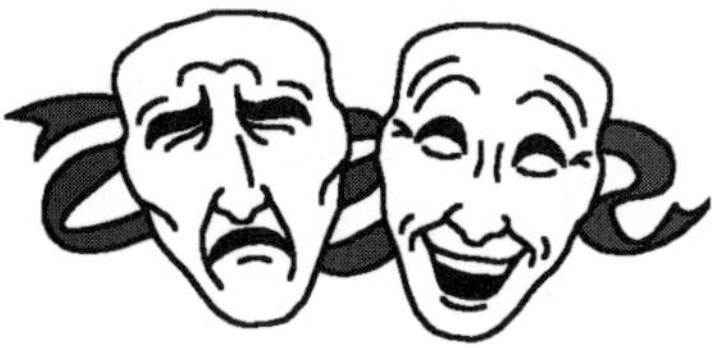

Everyone on your feet! This is our own standing ovation, to the people who contributed so generously to this book and to the dramas it describes.

To the central characters in *Standing Ovation*—Patricia Bower, Mary Sue Douglas, Vrenia Ivonoffski, Jan Livingston, Elaine Vanstone, and Ann Hampson—our wild and sustained applause. What you gave to *Handle with Care?*—creating and acting in it, and then reflecting with us on the whole messy process—formed the heart of this book.

We're grateful to Art Bochner for such a thorough embracing of our manuscript and our work, and for providing lots of warm encouragement and good editorial advice. Thanks to Carolyn Ellis for arranging for us to perform at the 2000 Couch Stone Symposium in St. Petersburg and for getting excited about *Handle with Care?* and to Mitch Allen for lending support and ensuring the project came to fruition.

Our sincere appreciation to the people who offered such careful attention to an earlier version of this book: Cheryl Badour, Kathryn Church, Ann Hampson, Ralph Osborne, and Elaine Vanstone. John Calderone and the production team at Rowman & Littlefield Publishers, Inc., hung in there when the formatting got tough, and the book is better for it.

Much enthusiastic clapping to the people whose generosity of time, energy, and spirit created *Handle with Care?*: Vrenia Ivonoffski,

Act II Studio's artistic director; the original crew of actors—Patricia Bower, Sandra Carter, Mary Sue Douglas, Phyllis Graham, Ruth Job, Jan Livingston, and Elaine Vanstone; the *Handle with Care?* script development group, which included the actors listed above along with Ann Hampson, Dvora Levinson, and Elaine Vayda; Fran Turner, project coordinator for *Handle with Care?* and *No Big Deal?*; the actors who joined along the way—Sandra Burley, Lou Cooper, Dave Cormack, Claudette Gareau, Barbara Haber, Sheila Miller, and Eugene Vayda; and the research team—Dr. Margaret Fitch, Marlene Greenberg, Ann Hampson, Barb Moore, Manon Labrecque, and Dr. Carol Sawka.

Many thanks to our hosts, and to everyone who attended performances of *Handle with Care?* in each of the communities we visited.[1] In Ontario: Barrie, Burlington, Chatham, Hamilton, Kingston, Kitchener-Waterloo, Little Current, London, Mississauga, Newmarket, North Bay, Oakville, Oshawa, Ottawa, Owen Sound, Peterborough, Richmond Hill, Sudbury, Thunder Bay, Timmins, Toronto, Whitby, Windsor, and Woodstock. For the National Tour (March–May, 2000): Surrey, Vancouver, and Victoria, British Columbia; Ottawa, Ontario; Yellowknife, Northwest Territories; Regina and Saskatoon, Saskatchewan; Brandon and Winnipeg, Manitoba; Fredericton, Moncton, and Saint John, New Brunswick; St. John's, Newfoundland; Halifax, Nova Scotia; Charlottetown and Summerside, Prince Edward Island; Calgary, Edmonton, and Red Deer, Alberta. In the United States, St. Petersburg, Florida, and Atlanta, Georgia.

And, finally, enthusiastic cheers for everyone involved in *No Big Deal?*—the research team, the script development group, and the actors.

It wouldn't have been what it was, or did what it did, without each one of you.

CHAPTER ONE
AND NOW INTRODUCING . . .

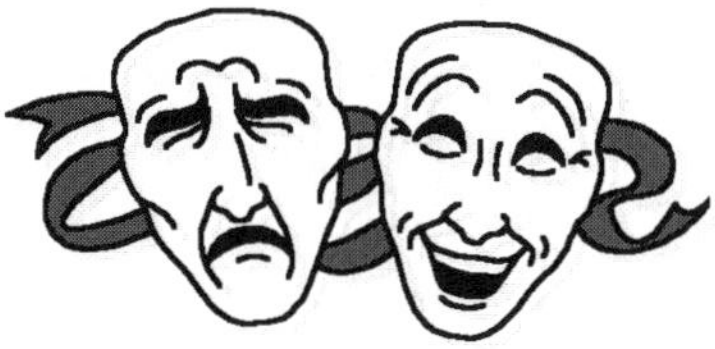

Seated on mismatched chairs in a room cluttered with props and discarded costumes, we introduced ourselves and began to talk. It was January 1998, and we were meeting for the first time: members of a research team based at Toronto Sunnybrook Regional Cancer Centre, actors from Act II Studio,[1] women with metastatic breast cancer, and women active in the breast cancer community. Our goal was to create a drama, working from focus group research conducted the previous year about the informational needs of women with metastatic breast cancer, and from a series of interviews with oncologists.

For several months, we explored what it means to have metastatic disease and what it means to provide oncological care to women with this diagnosis. We talked, told stories, exchanged copies of the research transcripts, cried, scribbled notes, argued, laughed, learned about body sculpture, and began to improvise key themes from the research. Over the summer, Act II Studio's artistic director, Vrenia Ivonoffski, gathered together the images and stretches of dialogue we had generated or selected from the transcripts and developed two formal scripts—one for health professional audiences, and one for the broader community. The entire group reviewed and reworked the scripts, attending to their resonance with the transcripts and with the knowledge we had created as a group. The scripts were further modified in response to feedback from test audiences of women with breast cancer and physicians. Multitudinous rehearsals ensued.

In October 1998, we launched *Handle with Care? Women Living with Metastatic Breast Cancer*, performing at Oncology Grand Rounds at the eight regional cancer centers in Ontario, and to public audiences in dozens of Ontario communities. Responding to unanticipated demand and success beyond our wildest hopes, we extended performances fifteen months beyond our original schedule and launched a national tour. By the time *Handle with Care?* ended in June 2000, we had performed before both community and health professional audiences in most major Canadian cities, and a handful of times in the United States. Countless local and regional media reports highlighted the drama's impact.[2] A radio program was broadcast nationally,[3] and a film documentary had been produced.[4] At our wrap-up party in June 2000, we celebrated almost 200 performances of *Handle with Care?*

This book tells the story of *Handle with Care? Living with Metastatic Breast Cancer*. In chapter 2, we locate our work within the burgeoning field of performance ethnography. Chapters 3, 4, and 5 trace the drama's development, recreating key moments—epiphanies, transitions—by layering together the reflections of cast members. Sections of the script that parallel our own learning about metastatic disease are integrated with the narrative.

In chapter 6, we recall our first quaking performances and begin to reflect on the responses of audience members to the drama. We explore the impact on cast members of their participation in *Handle with Care?* in chapters 7 and 8; chapter 8 also contains our discussion about what we would tell another group planning to embark on a project like ours and puts forward—albeit tentatively—some working principles for research-based drama.

In the following chapter, we document our "traveling and unraveling"—our national tour, and the various aspects of the project that began, over time, to fray at the edges. We also examine more carefully our relationships with people who witnessed the drama. As we performed *Handle with Care?* interactions with audience members—both formal and informal postperformance discussions as well as the unspoken back and forth between performers and viewers—taught us things, fed us joy and energy, and also surfaced discomfort and dissent. Sometimes the drama evoked strong feelings. Audience members often asked direct questions about how to handle a treatment decision or a relationship. As the group on stage, we didn't always know, or agree about, how to respond. Our struggle to find a place from which to hear and speak to people in audiences who engaged the drama with us is taken up in chapter 9. In chapter 10, we describe our final three performances.

Throughout *Standing Ovation*, Ross explains how his role as researcher has been unsettled and redefined by the *Handle with Care?* project. Periodically, he also draws on insights from another research-based drama, *No Big Deal?* about men with prostate cancer and their partners. As was the case with *Handle with Care?* the creative process towards a script for *No Big Deal?* started with

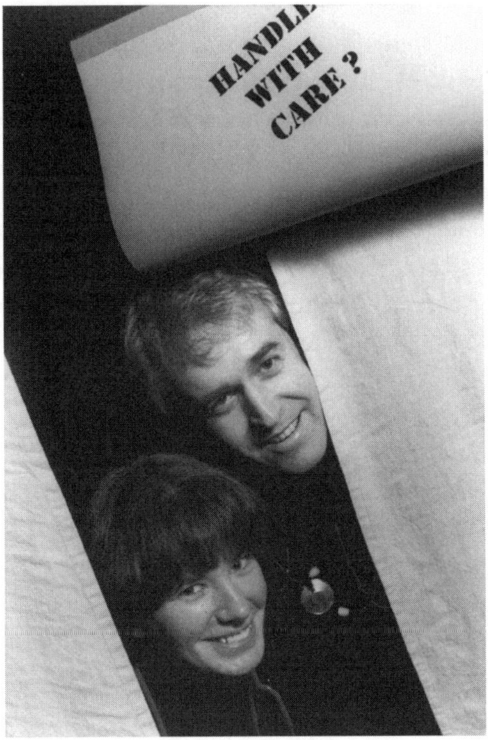

Ross and Christina

qualitative research undertaken by Ross and a team at the Toronto Sunnybrook Regional Cancer Centre. Men and their spouses were interviewed (separately) three times: before surgery to remove the men's prostates, two months after surgery, and a year later. The script development crew included members of the research team, men with prostate cancer and their spouses, and actors from Act II Studio. Ross examines points of comparison between the two dramas in chapter 8. The video that accompanies this book offers readers a chance to see each drama performed.

The narrative voices in *Standing Ovation* belong mainly to Ross and Christina. "Researcher Rants" and "Memorybank Dramas" inserted throughout the text allow the two of us to speak from various positions and with various voices. When, as part of an improvisation exercise, a member of the script development group went off on a passionate tear about some issue or another, Vrenia declared this a "rant" for the purposes of cataloguing it in her growing stash of script material. While our Researcher Rants sometimes fail to sustain the energy the term promises (descending into "reflections" and "musings"), we like the implied momentum, and the gesture towards distinction from traditional research discourse. Margaret Laurence, in her novel *The Diviners* (1974), used "Memorybank Movie" to mark sections of text that drew images or experiences from the past into her present-day narrative. We use Memorybank Dramas in a similar way; the device also makes space for us each to speak more personally in the text.

In weaving this story together, we draw on our own experiences as researchers and, later, as actors in the drama. We also rely on extensive notes taken during the early meetings of the group and interviews conducted with the people intimately involved in *Handle with Care?* Over time, we recorded several conversations with the women with metastatic disease, with a handful of the actors and Act II Studio's artistic director, with each other and the rest of the research team, trying to generate a range of experiences and perspectives on the process of linking research to drama. Although we would have wished to include the voices of each person whose energy and commitment informed *Handle with Care?* for the sake of clarity we draw mainly from interviews with:

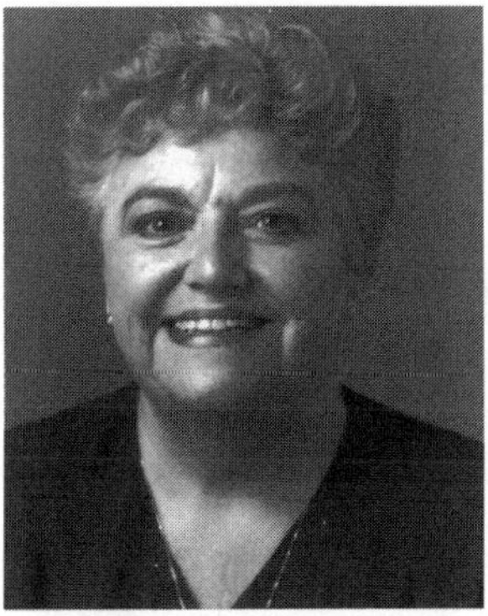

Patricia: an actor and breast cancer survivor—the little, laughing, determinedly hopeful one

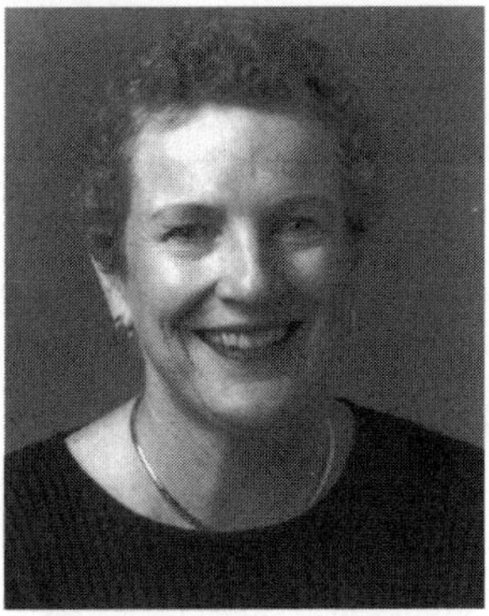

Mary Sue: AKA "the diva," a woman active in cancer support and cancer center policy, and living with metastatic breast cancer

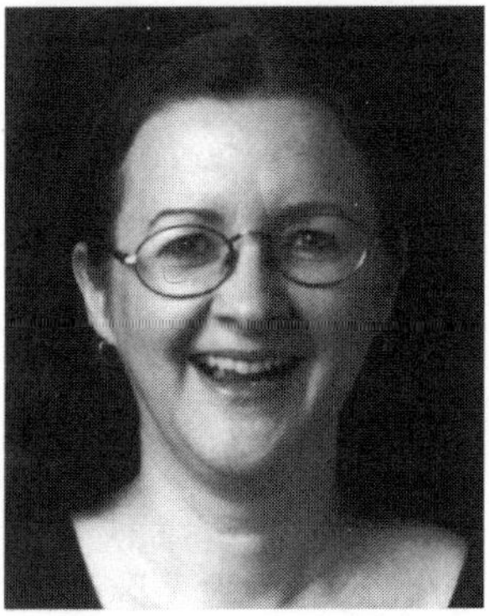

Vrenia: Act II Studio's artistic director, an anarchist, creative genius, and proponent of the value of panic

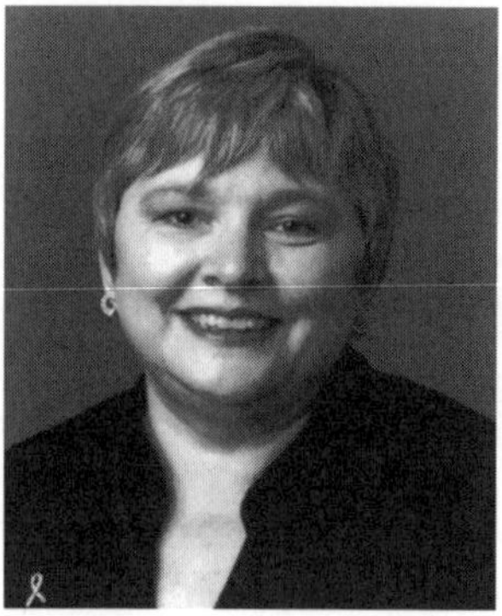

Jan: Orillia's local hero, the media darling, educator, communicator, a woman living with metastatic breast cancer

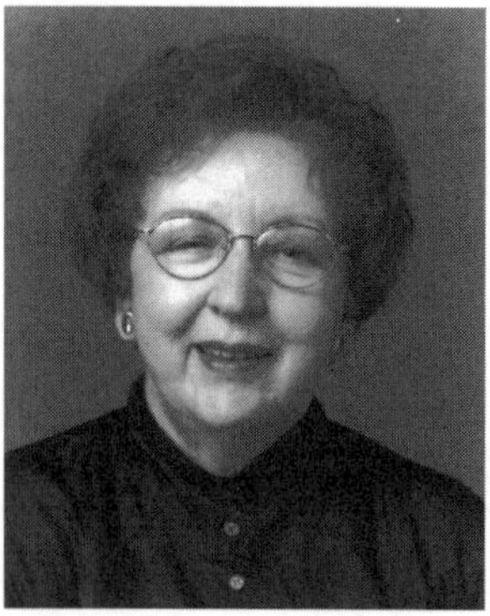

Elaine: an actor and retired nurse, attentive to all the logistical and human details, whose proper demeanor belies a cunning wit

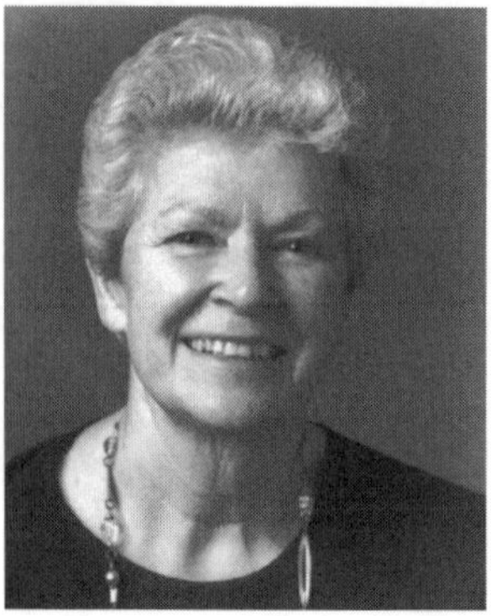

Ann: the member of the research team who conducted the original focus groups with women living with metastatic breast cancer; someone who has herself experienced a breast cancer diagnosis, and the "wise woman" of the group

❋

Linking social science research to drama is heady, dangerous work. Like many others in the fledgling field of performance ethnography, we are interested in the complicated process of producing "messy texts" (Marcus 1994)—critical, experimental forms of ethnography that

> confront the problem that ethnography, which is centrally interested in the creativity of social action through imagination, narrativity, and performance, has usually been produced though an analytic imagination that in contrast is impoverished. (Marcus 1994, 567)

In a messy text, the object of study is not assimilated into analytic categories; on the contrary, such texts resist analytic closure, affirming that knowledge is always partial and always being negotiated with audiences. Messy texts focus on the stories people tell to make sense of turning points in their lives, incorporating many voices and privileging none (Denzin 1997). Attending to the intersections between private troubles and shared culture (Mills 1959), they represent those intersections in imaginative, evocative ways (Denzin 1997). Messy texts expand the relevance of qualitative research (e.g., Conquergood 1991; Ellis and Bochner 1992; Jackson 1989; Marcus 1994; McCall and Becker 1990; Mienczakowski 1996a; Pelias 1999; Trinh 1991; Walstrom 1996).

The touchstones against which experimental ethnographies are assessed differ from those of traditional research products. Here, the capacity to enable emotional engagement is crucial (Ellis and Flaherty 1992), as is the work's potential to move people to moral action (Denzin 1997). The goal is to bring "felt news" from one world to another (Denzin 1997).

Handle with Care? and *No Big Deal?* began, for the most part, as traditionally conceived qualitative research projects. Conversant with debates in the field, the research team acknowledged that such research has its own "messiness." We believe that interviews and focus groups are sites and sources of multiple interpretative acts. We know that writing up qualitative studies often involves knitting together quite disparate threads such that they seem to form a coherent analytic whole, inserted neatly under this theme or that.

We agreed, then, that the research component of this project had itself been complicated, untidy, and occasionally angst ridden. But having worked through this particular stage, we felt fairly confident about our capacity to articulate a reasonable range of realities around women's informational needs when they are living with metastatic breast cancer, and around the experiences of men with prostate cancer and their spouses. Trusting in the transcripts and our initial analysis of them, we entered the creative process. And found complication on a grand scale, messiness writ large.

Neck-deep and floundering, we released our grip on familiar notions of truth telling and moved to embrace a more evocative epistemology (Denzin 1997). *Handle with Care?* and *No Big Deal?* are pastiches of voices and gestures—voices and gestures explored, debated, agonized and argued over, and, finally, settled and staged. Linked to, but not bound by, the research transcripts, the dramas are infused with the energy of our connections to one another and the multiple, shifting realities of living with illness.

Researcher Rant: August 2000: Ross

Looking back, I'm incredulous at the gall I had to launch into this project with so little clue of what I was doing. But I have to admit it's typical. For me, to think too carefully from the outset, to line up all the possible barriers and review them, to immerse myself in the literature written by all my brighter and more talented peers—this immobilizes me. Sometimes acting before thinking things through gets me in trouble; sometimes it works really well. But it's never an easy route. *Handle with*

Care? has taken me on a roller coaster ride I could never have anticipated.

One of my motivations with this project was to take the opportunity to write creatively, to produce a script. It took me a while to see how unprepared to achieve this goal I was. Publishing for academic journals—at least the kind for which I had been writing—was no kind of preparation for script writing. I knew nothing about staging and was oblivious to the nuances of visual presentation. For too many years, I have been held captive by written text.

Like others involved with the project, I wrote a few pieces of the script. But Vrenia was the major architect of *Handle with Care?* For our second research-based production, *No Big Deal?* about prostate cancer issues, we have cowritten the script in roughly equal measure. But it has been clear that I am the apprentice.

Other social scientists experimenting with drama have advantages I don't possess. Jim Mienczakowski, for instance, a pioneer in ethnodrama, combines ethnography skills with a theater background. But researchers newly exploring the dramatic sphere would likely benefit, as I have, from working with colleagues experienced in the expressive arts.

❋

Our aim in *Standing Ovation* is to create what John Van Maanen calls an "impressionist tale," a tale that draws readers into the active process of *Handle with Care?* with us. Such tales are representational means of "cracking open the culture and the fieldworker's way of knowing it so both can be jointly examined" (Van Maanen 1988, 102). In our context, each of the people involved in *Handle with Care?* was a kind of fieldworker, struggling to both understand and represent the meanings of living with metastatic breast cancer.

The epistemological aim of an impressionist tale is to "braid the knower with the known" (Van Maanen 1988, 103). When the *Handle with Care?* crew first met, the stacks of paper the research team presented—transcripts from focus groups with women who had metastatic disease and from interviews with oncologists—were to most of us just that: stacks of paper. Over the course of the drama's creation, the voices in those texts were made audible. The women's voices, the physician's voices, wove through our conversations as a group.

As we worked together on the drama, each person in the *Handle with Care?* troupe moved into and out of the spaces occupied by women living with metastatic disease. We came to know Mary Sue and Jan, the two women in the group with advanced breast cancer, and they came to know us. By the time we took our last bows, the entire troupe was intimately connected.

Laughing and tearful, audiences in lecture halls and community centers across the country braided into the drama as well, creating and recreating the myriad meanings of metastatic disease and the myriad ways we can respond to the illness—as women living with it, and as friends, colleagues, and supporters.

❋

We say this is an impressionist tale. Yet if you turn the page, you'll find a literature review—a tale of sorts, but not exactly what Van Maanen had in mind.

You may want to watch the video included with this book now, to have a sense of the dramas themselves. The story behind the dramas begins in chapter 3.

CHAPTER TWO

SOCIAL SCIENCE MEETS PERFORMANCE

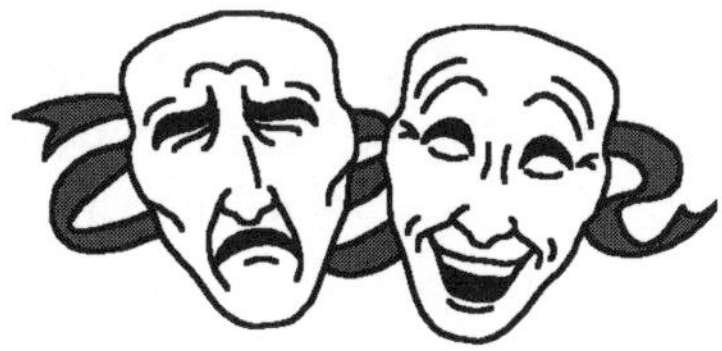

The current alliance between social science and performance can be traced to many sources, its history told in a variety of ways (see Conquergood 1991; Denzin 1997; McCall 2000). Social science tellings of the history usually begin with the work of sociologist Erving Goffman. Four decades ago, Goffman introduced the metaphor of the stage into sociological discourse, highlighting the ways people seek to foster and control the impression of self that others have of them (Goffman 1963; Williams 1987).

"Backstage" is the space in which, according to Goffman, we review our performances, change costumes, and plan our next roles and scenes. Later theorists contested Goffman's notion of a "backstage" free from the decisions and machinations of acting. In this view, one never leaves the stage; each theatrical exit "becomes simultaneously an entrance onto another stage" (Conquergood 1992, 92). Performance events are not (merely) what we do for public viewing. Planned and not, they construct identity, and they are "the very stuff and heart of culture" (Conquergood 1992, 84).

Attending to ethnography as both a method of social science research and a genre of social science text, Conquergood credits Victor Turner's (1986) conceptualization of performance for shifting ethnography away from the assumptions of colonialist and objectivist social science and initiating the second movement of performance. Turner "subversively redefined the fundamental terms of discussion in ethnography by defining humankind as *homo performans*, humanity as performer, a culture-inventing, social-performing, self-making and self-transforming creature" (Conquergood 1991, 187).

If objectivist social science holds that self and culture are stable entities, amenable to singular, authoritative explanations, the paradigm Turner proposed—bolstered by the philosophy of language—holds that culture circulates through us; we enact culture even in the most daily of performances. In an objectivist framework, people and culture "are," and researchers, looking carefully, perceive and map our universal patterns. Now, people "do" culture, making and remaking and changing identities and cultures, in relation to particular and shifting local and historical circumstances.

In the third movement Conquergood identifies, performance becomes inflected with poststructuralism and focuses attention on personal and social struggle. "Performative" then refers to those discursive acts that "insinuate, interrupt, interrogate and antagonize powerful master discourses" (Conquergood 1992, 84).

Ethnographers, and social scientists more broadly, have taken up these various conceptualizations of performance in a range of ways, exploring, for instance, the implications of a performance framework for doing fieldwork, and interpreting fieldwork notes (Conquergood 1991). Pelias writes poetically about performance, both in its daily and formal meanings, as a way of knowing (Pelias 1999). Conquergood also reflects on—and notes a relative lack of academic attention to—the possibilities of performance as a complementary form of disseminating research findings (Conquergood 1991). *Standing Ovation* explores performance both as a means of engaging with stories gathered through qualitative research methods, and as a vehicle for "publishing" the knowledge generated from that engagement.

Among those involved in the performance of research findings, McCall distinguishes the approaches and aims of people who "come from" ethnography and those who "come from" theater or performance studies. In her brief history of performance ethnography (McCall 2000), McCall notes that the late 1980s and early 1990s were boundary-crossing times, with sociologists beginning to turn ethnographic field notes into performances, and theater artists and academics in performance studies producing or adapting ethnographies in order to perform them. She describes her own work with Becker and Morris, in which they translated formal interviews with seventy actors, directors, and theater workers into performance pieces that described career issues and the social organization of theater communities (Becker, McCall, and Morris 1989; McCall and Becker 1990).

McCall (2000) contrasts these scripts with the efforts of theater artists and performance studies academics, particularly Emilie Beck's *The Work of Talk*, adapted from an article by Marianne Paget (Paget 1983); Della Pollock's adaptation (1990) of Hall's study *Like a Family: The Making of a Southern Cotton Mill World* (Hall, Leloudis, et al. 1987); and Anna Deavere Smith's *Fires in the Mirror* (1993) and *Twilight* (1994); and also with her own later work (McCall 1993).

She notes that while theater artists and people in performance studies were informed by the history of performance art and experimental theater, the performance work of sociologists was very much text based: "There was a story, the words did mean something, and there were very few images to listen to" (McCall 2000). The sociologists performed using scripts, without costumes or props, and with limited movement on the stage.

In "Performance Science"—a script published in the journal *Social Problems* in 1990—McCall and Becker describe their use in performance of large chunks of verbatim quotations from their field notes "with only minimal interpretation" (122). A lot of data gets communicated, they claimed, and

MICHAL: The selection and arrangement of the stories embodies a rudimentary analysis.
HOWIE: Maybe as much as anyone really needs.
MICHAL: And, perhaps more important, information about mood and emotion, as well as events and attitudes, gets transmitted. (McCall and Becker 1990, 122)

In continuing to muse on what happens when ethnography is performed, Becker ("Howie" above) describes speaking the sentence, "casting really is a problem" out loud, and confronting

> something that everyone learns as a kid—that you can alter the meaning of a sentence by changing which words you emphasize. . . . And having done that, I lost my innocence forever. From then on, I knew—could never forget—that whether I emphasized "casting," "really is," or "problem," whether I thought about it or not, the choice was not 'natural' and obvious. It was a real choice that I could have made some other way. (McCall and Becker 1990, 125)

Each rendering of the sentence pointed to different analytic pathways, different ways of conceptualizing the "real" problem. The point that McCall and Becker make from the interchange and from the moment of Becker's lost innocence is that performing a text can be a way of understanding the substance of a topic. Certainly this was true in *Handle with Care?* and *No Big Deal?* as we made decisions about the tone and emphasis of each scene, each line in the script. The tone *Handle with Care?* finally achieved emerged in many ways from the shifts that occurred within the script development group as we learned about metastatic breast cancer and came to know Mary Sue and Jan, shifts we describe in chapters 3 and 7.

Yet perhaps more critically, Becker also points to one of the key axes upon which performance ethnography, emerging from both the world of theater and the world of social science, turns: the relationship between the performed text and what went before—that is, the data-gathering situation, and before (and beyond) that, the lived experience.

At least two impulses emerge from the choice Becker is required to make about how the line will be spoken: an impulse back to "the data," and an impulse towards the audience. Return to the tape, the interview situation, recall the focus group; or, shift focus, and imagine what you want the piece to say or do to an audience.

In *Handle with Care?* and *No Big Deal?* we teetered between these two impulses, alternately anxious to make sure the dramas "presented" the interview material in some truthful way and wanting to have it evoke something in the people who would—someday—maybe—witness the performance.

Other people had teetered here before us, of course. Denzin divides the social science engagement with performance into two broad categories: that which employs a performance science model and that which is consistent with "a critical, postmodern, performance aesthetic" (Denzin 1997, 113). We will consider first the performance science legacy.

Performance scientists translate field notes and field texts in a literal way, maintaining a deep commitment to the data-gathering site and its original meanings (Denzin 1997). In this tradition, Denzin includes Jackson (1993), Paget (1993), Stucky (1993), and Becker et al. (Becker, McCall, and Morris 1989); we might also include McCall (1993). Some people "from theater" use approaches similar to those explicitly named "performance science;" see, for instance, the history of verbatim theater (Paget 1987); also Smith (1993; 1994); Beck's work, as described by Paget (1993); and, recently, *The Laramie Project* (Kaufman 2000). The difference here is that theater artists, even as they locate the source of their performance in a data-gathering situation and in some cases adhere quite rigorously to field notes and field texts, often have an eye to the audience in ways social scientists usually do not (see, for instance, Paget 1987, 324).

Many adherents to the "performance science" model ensure that performances are intimately bound to the data-gathering site by attending carefully not only to the words spoken in interview situations but also to the sound of those words. Stucky (1993), for instance, focuses on the aesthetics of natural performances, asking the people who perform the work to listen to recorded conversations for details of intonation and voice quality.

When McCall and her colleagues staged *Not Just a Farmer and Not Just a Farm Wife*, "we were not acting; we were simply reading aloud the traces of a conversation among ourselves and four women farmers" (McCall 1993, 430). McCall seeks to minimize the amount of interpretive work required by performers by transcribing the sounds of words, and pauses, and transferring these to the script.

McCall likens her current approach to that of Anna Deavere Smith, who undertakes interviews with people involved in particular events and bases the script entirely on this interview material. *Twilight: Lost Angeles, 1992* is, says Smith, "the product of my search for the character of Los Angeles in the wake of the initial Rodney King verdict" (Smith, cited in McCall 2000, 430). Smith's aim is to create the illusion of being another person by reenacting something they had said *as they had said it* (Smith cited in McCall 2000, 431, emphasis in original).

Verbatim theater, as well, maintains a scrupulous link to the interview, while explicitly refusing the notion that actors are "impersonating" people who took part in those interviews (Paget 1987, 332). Substantial elements of the production consist of transcripts from interviews. The source material "becomes the true protagonist in the drama" (Paget 1987, 318).

Derek Paget traces the history of verbatim theater in a British context, locating its origins in radio documentaries of the 1950s and the documentary film movement in the two decades prior. In Paget's article, Cheeseman[1] describes a "puritanism" about the use of oral history to make plays, a meticulousness about how the material is collected, transcribed, and annotated.

Kaufman's *The Laramie Project* emerged from a search similar to the one Smith undertook in Los Angeles, and was conducted in a manner congruent with the verbatim theater process Paget describes. Kaufman began from the conviction that the brutal murder of gay college student Matthew Shepard in Laramie, Wyoming, illuminated key cultural struggles. In the course of speculating about how theater might contribute to national dialogue on current events, he came across an essay by Brecht. In *The Street Scene*, Brecht uses as a model the situation of "an eyewitness describing to a collection of people how a traffic accident took place" (Brecht, cited in Kaufman 2000, 1). Upon this model, Brecht builds a theory about "epic theater." Reading *The Street Scene* suggested an approach and conceptual framework to Kaufman, and he and members of his Tectonic Theatre Project traveled to Laramie. Over almost a dozen visits, company members interviewed more than 200 people, transcribed the interviews, and presented them to the rest of the troupe.

In the face of a growing volume of material, Kaufman created a writers' group to assist him in the rich but difficult process of sorting through the transcripts and selecting what would be in the play. Reducing such a mass of source material "to some sort of viable theatrical shape" is, in the words of one verbatim theater director, "a bit of a head bending experience" (Paget 1987, 323).

Head bending indeed. Although the introduction of a formally trained researcher into the mix might have eased the strain of wrapping their minds around the transcripts, neither Kaufman nor the practitioners of verbatim theater appear to have sought such assistance. Their decision to go it alone parallels the approach currently undertaken by many social scientists who are writing scripts and performing them with nary an artistic director in sight. Although interesting and valuable work is clearly emerging with each field working in relative isolation from the other, we would still advocate for interdisciplinary and intersectoral exchange. Collaborative arts-based social science is flourishing in education colleges. Such work, among its many other virtues, mitigates against the spectacle of the arts becoming a site of imperialist expansion by researchers (or vice versa).

In our case, a certain "reduction" of the source material had taken place when Ross and the research team at Sunnybrook completed a thematic analysis of the focus group and interview transcripts. Ross listed those themes on a sheet of paper distributed to everyone involved in the project. In the early days of *Handle with Care?* when the script development group seemed to be launching in various disparate directions, Ross was determined that these themes set the boundaries for what would be included in the drama. "I'll be stubborn about it.

Like we're not going to do something that isn't on that sheet, absolutely not."

We were not, however, stubborn about the transcripts themselves. Ross struggled a bit with this in the early days of *Handle with Care?* A significant source of his inspiration for research-based theater was the work of Jim Mienczakowski and his colleagues in Australia, whose "ethnodrama" "adheres to the principles of a formal and recognizable ethnographic research methodology, above and beyond the artistic demands of aesthetics, in its attempts to produce cultural critique" (Mienczakowski 1999, 157).[2]

As part of his commitment to validity, Mienczakowski relies primarily on the actual words and constructions offered by contributors to the research; in *Busting*, for instance, a drama about alcoholism, almost 90 percent of the script is transcribed words of study respondents (Mienczakowski and Morgan 1994, 80). Ross wondered if we shouldn't do this as well, with *Handle with Care?* But Vrenia, influenced by training from Jacques Lecoq, advocated a different approach.

Lecoq identified a "circular response between actors and audience" (Brady 1999, 3) and emphasized (as did Vrenia) using and training the body in particular ways (see chapter 5). In Lecoq's vision, the actor is not an instrument (as is claimed in, for instance, verbatim theater) nor an interpreter, but a creator. The actor must understand the topic, approaching the material in a spirit of inquiry (Brady 1999, 2), and, as Vrenia said, "internalizing." Internalizing may involve a close reading of the transcripts, and might also involve listening to tape-recorded interviews, but neither is sufficient.

"*Internalizing* means processing material on a very subjective level," said Vrenia, "absorbing the experience shared by the women in the focus groups. Trying to confront our own fears openly in the presence of Mary Sue and Jan—and responding to them without seeking safety." In addition to reaching "backwards" to the data-gathering situation and "forwards" to the audience, then, we also reached sideways to one another, and inside ourselves, as we describe in chapter 4.

A drama that emerges from such a process is very much a negotiated settlement, a collective achievement. The knowledge foregrounded in our script development process emerged from, but was not contained by, what was said in the transcripts or how it was said. And that is perhaps what distinguishes *Handle with Care?* from the performance science tradition, and aligns it more closely with what Denzin calls improvisational ethnodrama. Again, the issue is the status of the performance text as it relates to the data-gathering experience. "Improvisational, ethnodrama texts fundamentally transform that experience . . . improvisational ethnodrama alters and changes the field text, producing composite characters, emphasizing multiple tellings of the same event, and shifting concern away from verisimilitude toward dramatic reinterpretation and cultural critique" (Denzin 1997, 100). Here, Denzin does not use "improvisation" to refer to a performance that is improvised in the moment (though he also discusses this (see Denzin 1997, 123); rather, he advocates for scripts which "improvise on" data gathered in interviews and focus groups.

Emilie Beck's *The Work of Talk* was first published by Marianne Paget (1983) as a research article, an analysis of a series of exchanges between a physician and a woman with cancer. Beck moved Paget's article onto the stage almost verbatim. The performance that emerged, Paget argues, was almost entirely "factual," faithful to the written analysis. The key "fictional" element lay in Beck's decision to make Cancer the narrator of the drama. "Here is one of the conundrums of the performance," Paget writes. "The performance made fantastic some of the facts in order to state them" (Paget 1983, 32). From the framework of improvisational ethnodrama, Beck's decision is not a conundrum: it is the very point of "an evocative epistemology that performs rather than represents the world" (Denzin 1997, 115). Chapter 5 of this book describes some of our own departures from naturalistic representation, our attempts to "perform" something of people's experiences living with serious illness.

Part of Denzin's commitment to an improvisational approach hearkens back to Conquergood's critique of the "old" ethnography.

Natural performance texts, seeking to capture an objective reality (asserting, for instance, that "actual facts" are being presented, reminding the viewer that "real people" spoke these words) can appear very much like authorized tellings. In creating the appearance of a singular truth, such tales "reproduce the pull of realism and run the risk of not criticizing what they reproduce" (Denzin 1997, 114).[3] From Denzin's perspective, the researcher's goal is not to put forward something that "looks like the truth" but rather to contrast multiple verisimilitudes, multiple truths. Even more critically, though, such work involves a commitment to morally move readers and viewers. For audiences to understand what one party in a dialogue—the researcher—has come to understand, the researcher's text (the article, document, poem, drama) must offer audience members a way "to enter into the parts and spaces of listener and speaker. Only in this way will it be possible . . . to bring to (and take from) this text the same depth of understanding and sympathy that is brought to their own experience" (Denzin 1997, 39). Chapter 5 of *Standing Ovation* documents how *Handle with Care?* performs the multiple and shifting realities of women's relationship to information when they are living with metastatic breast cancer. We also examine the ways the drama interfaces with cultural critique and problematizes "right action" in relation to someone who is seriously ill.

Scholars of performance ethnography often attend carefully to the negotiation over meaning that occurs between actors and audiences, and some examine the interpretive interface between research transcripts and a performance text. Few describe the kind of script development process we undertook, itself a dynamic back and forth between multiple players and multiple sources of knowledge. Each of us, in her or his own way, took in the transcripts, struggled with the feelings evoked by the women's words, and took on the task of representation. Each scene in *Handle with Care?*—its image, its tone—was "tested" in the moment of its creation against Mary Sue's and Jan's lived experience of the illness. And all of the voices—the voices in the transcripts, the researchers' voices, the actors', the director's, the voices of the two women with metastatic breast cancer—eventually became resonant, in every moment of the drama.

Denzin claims that improvisational performance texts are the "single most powerful way for ethnography to recover yet interrogate the meanings of lived experience" (Denzin 1997, 95). We liked that line when we read it. We hadn't much idea what we were doing when we plunged into the world of research-based theater, but Denzin sure made it sound promising.

CHAPTER THREE

THE MEANING OF "METASTATIC"

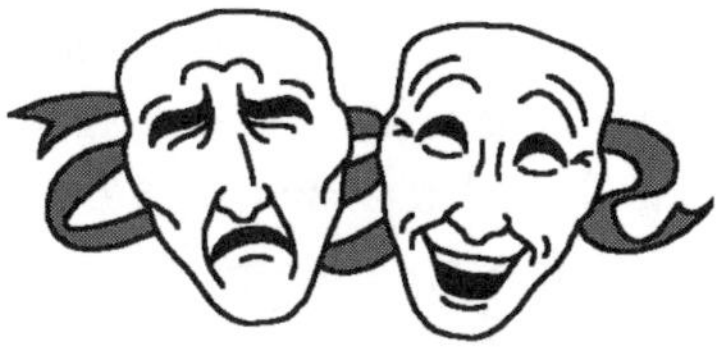

Memorybank Drama: March 1997: Ross

It is not easy to retrace my steps, to say how it all started. Just before I decided to write the initial proposal for our research-based drama project, I was reading Laurel Richardson's chapter in *The Handbook of Qualitative Research* about writing as a form of inquiry. She wrote, "It seems foolish at best, and narcissistic and wholly self-absorbed at worst, to spend months or years doing research that ends up not being read and not making a difference to anything but the author's career" (Richardson 1994, 517). These words resurfaced the familiar doubt that I've felt through the years about the social usefulness of my own research work—despite ongoing attempts to be relevant and applied in my approach.

In the same chapter, Richardson referred to writing scripts for theater as a possible vehicle for presenting research results. I was intrigued. I had been thinking about trying to write a script for a while but had seen that possibility unfolding on my personal time, not related to work. Frustrated creativity has been a thread in my life; passion for the expressive arts links backwards in time to the unfinished novel in my desk drawer, to the binder filled with my unpublished poems. I was also wearing thin from a certain type of academic productivity. I found myself sitting at my desk, thinking that if I had to write one more paper for journal publication I would be sick, literally. I was tired of reviewers expecting me to speak less plainly, more abstractly, telling me to take the little jokes out of my manuscripts—tired of needing to conform to the torpid, deadly serious style of academic writing.

So, turning to drama came from two places. It represented a new pathway to try to make a difference in the world through social science research and it was also an outlet, a desperate reaching towards balance, an attempt to disrupt and lighten the weighty darkness of professional academic life.

My sudden interest in linking research to drama quickly found a context within ongoing work. Our research group at the Toronto Sunnybrook Regional Cancer Centre had been meeting regularly to reflect together on some very evocative transcripts from focus groups we had conducted with women with metastatic breast cancer. The material was so rich it seemed to cry out for fuller exposure than would be provided by the article I was drafting for a professional cancer journal (Gray, Greenberg, Fitch, Sawka, Hampson, Labrecque, and Moore 1998). And there was a funding deadline that just happened to be coming up at the Canadian Breast Cancer Foundation.

So I did what I have done countless times before, dashed off a proposal, hastily cobbling together a partnership with various organizations. We proposed to take the results of our study of women with metastatic breast cancer, and of a companion study with medical oncologists treating breast cancer patients, and use them to create a dramatic production. We would take it on tour. I sent the grant proposal off and turned my attention to the next one.

I sometimes wonder if I would have taken the first step towards developing *Handle with Care?* had I known all the challenges that awaited. I entered the field blissfully unaware of what we were in for.

❋

Memorybank Drama: March 1997: Christina

I remember the day Ross called me about the funding application he had drafted, to create a drama from research transcripts. At the time, I was coordinator of a provincial network of breast cancer self-help groups. Ross had phoned to see if I would write a letter of support for his funding request. We talked very briefly and he faxed the proposal over.

Ross and I had worked together the previous year. The focus group transcripts he was referring to had provided the launching point for an annotated bibliography of resources I had created with the research team at Sunnybrook, called *Living with Metastatic Breast Cancer*. I had enjoyed working with him, and had a sense of him as a decent sort of person, intelligent, thoughtful, respectful of the work that women did in support groups. I hadn't pegged him as the dramatic type.

Reading the proposal was delicious. I remember thinking the idea was utterly brilliant. There was so little available in the breast cancer community that reflected the experiences of women with advanced disease. I wrote an effusive letter of support.

The possibilities of drama were exciting to me, and also, in an odd sense, generated a kind of relief. So much of what we—our organization and the myriad others across the country—had created to respond to the struggles and questions of women with breast cancer was text based. Some of it was excellent, of course. But there was always that gap, that disconnection: on the one hand, the embodied reality of a woman anxiously rehearsing a treatment decision, or looking for the first time at her mastectomy scar, or plunging into her first support group meeting. On the other, the reassuring prose of our pamphlets, booklets, manuals. I had the sense of things connecting, with a drama. Things escaping. Becoming more true.

Not long after I wrote that letter, I was accepted into a doctoral program in Public Health Sciences at the University of Toronto. Over the summer, I started thinking about my future in a different way, wondering how I might begin to bolster my credentials as a researcher in the world. "Why don't you call Ross?" my partner suggested. "He might have some research-type work you could do." So I did, thinking I might do some interviews with people with cancer, or code some data. Ross promised to keep me in mind for any contract work that appeared.

And then, in November, Ross heard from Canadian Breast Cancer Foundation: his proposal had been approved. He asked if I'd consider coming on board to document the process of linking research to drama, and to help organize the community performances of the play. I said yes. Unaware. Blissfully so.

❋

It is January 1998. People filter into the building at 55 Gould Street on the Ryerson University campus in Toronto, unfolding from coats and scarves. Eventually we seem to have a quorum: a few researchers, several actors, one artistic director, two women with metastatic breast cancer.

Ross welcomes everyone and launches into the task. "We want to take what our researchers learned from focus groups with women who have metastatic breast cancer and create a play. We hope to reach health professionals at Grand Rounds, and women with breast cancer, and their families and friends, in the community."

He takes a substantial stack of papers from his bag, lands them heavily on a chair. "The transcripts may be overwhelming," he cautions. "The article we wrote"—another, smaller stack of paper—"summarizes the issues. Our main interest," he continues, "is to make sure that the women's perspectives are reflected in the play. Health professionals will pay more attention if we stay closely linked to the research. Does anyone have any questions?"

It all sounded so straightforward then. But the process of creating *Handle with Care?* was anything but neat and linear. One of our first obstacles was a word: the word "metastatic."

When Ross had met with Vrenia to discuss the creation of a partnership between Sunnybrook and Act II Studio, Vrenia had explained that translating the research material into a theatrical production would require a group effort. According to her vision, each person would come to some understanding of the intimate concerns of women living with metastatic breast cancer, and the script would emerge from this process.

This approach assumes that the people involved understand the basic medical realities of metastatic breast cancer. It became apparent at our first meeting, however, that "metastatic" was a new—and meaningless—word to several members of the theater group. Their frames of reference were the images and stories of women with breast cancer that pervade our culture: images and stories of heroic survivors, battling medical incompetence, visualizing themselves well.

At our second meeting, one actor asked Jan what it was like to have lost a breast and how her husband had reacted. (Jan replied that she had sliced the husband off before the breast.) Another declared that Mary Sue's and Jan's positive approach would see them through. One woman suggested we title the drama *We Shall Survive*.

Memorybank Drama: February 1998: Christina

It was like one of those excruciating movie scenes where the whole family is gathered around for a holiday dinner and there is an enormous unspoken truth, a disruptive truth, a truth that two or three of them know and the rest don't. The ones who know glance at one another, desperate to speak, to have the truth spoken. The rest are passing the gravy.

I hate those movies. I agonize for everybody at the table.

> I wanted to stop our meeting and say, "This is all wrong. This is not about losing a breast. This is not about 'getting beyond' this disease." And yet every way I tried to formulate the words in my head they came out brutal. I barely knew Mary Sue; I had no idea what she believed or knew about metastatic disease, or what she was prepared to hear. And who was I to speak up? I was supposed to be the research assistant, the one taking notes. I stewed about what Ross would think if I leapt in. So I sat, probably looking fairly calm, but utterly tied in knots inside.

❋

Confusion around the word "metastatic" quickly became awkward for nearly everyone. In a flurry of conversations and phone calls between meetings, various interventions were proposed.

Finally, it is decided: Marg, a member of the research team, will give "the cancer lecture" at the next meeting. She brings diagrams of cell structure and charts about life expectancy. "When cells break off from the original tumor and start to grow somewhere else, this is considered a metastases," she explains. "If growth is unchecked, cancer takes over the body. Metastatic disease is likely to shorten one's life."

People listen attentively. Then someone asks if men get breast cancer. "Yes," Ross says, "but we didn't try to deal with that in our research." Another actor wonders if women in small communities are informed about breast reconstruction. A few people make reassuring noises about how much better cancer treatments are these days.

Perhaps the drama will give women a chance to vent their anger at not being taken seriously by their doctors, one woman says. Others chime in with stories of caring physicians. Vrenia wonders if we might have a musical piece in the drama, about patients trying to get their questions answered.

We swing back to the conversation about metastatic disease, approaching and retreating from its distinction from a primary breast cancer diagnosis.

"It's the same enemy, isn't it?" someone asks. "It's different this time," replies Mary Sue. "When it's a primary diagnosis, you hope to be on the one end of Marg's chart—the 80 percent survival line. With metastatic disease, you're not on that line."

Jan tells the group about planning for a friend's fiftieth birthday party. "I was thinking, 'Damn! I'm going to die before my fiftieth,'" she says ruefully. "It puts an end on things," agrees Mary Sue.

And yet the discussion shifts again, away from the seriousness of metastatic disease, of a primary cancer advancing incurably to another part of the body. Someone makes reference to a play she saw about a man who was dying as if it has nothing to do with us, as if dying were irrelevant to what we are struggling with in this room.

Memorybank Drama: February 1998: Ross

I was not happy. I was angry that it had come to this. I thought I'd been clear.

When I had sat with Vrenia in that coffee shop, I'd said it straight out: "Think about these women as you would your friends with AIDS. Barring the miraculous, cure is not in the picture." I'd assumed this was the message that would get passed on to the volunteer actors she would invite to participate in the project. Months later, Vrenia had no memory of this conversation, only that she hadn't liked my serious, uptight manner. And she admitted that she'd been terrified by the idea of the project, not wanting to know more about breast cancer.

So now, I would have to do it: I would have to read out mortality statistics to the script development group. I was not happy. Over the years of sitting with people with cancer, I've learned how vulnerable they are to discouragement and despair. It's as if the work of being ill takes everything that they have, leaving little psychic energy left to deal with whatever else comes along. Whether or not they speak it, most are traumatized, casting about for anything that will ease the terror.

When my friend Jim was waiting for his bone marrow transplant for leukemia, eight different health professionals warned him that the treatment would be incredibly difficult. Maybe, just maybe, it served a purpose for him to hear that message once—in the unlikely event that he might have believed it would be a breeze, or made plans to go scuba diving or play golf in the days or weeks post-treatment. But he certainly didn't need to be told more than once. So it is with survival statistics. Women with metastatic breast cancer, unless they've managed a rare type of denial, know that it's serious stuff. To throw the bleak statistics into a room is to assault them, hurt them, set them back, make them draw deep on their resources to once again climb out of the darkness and carry on.

I called Mary Sue, whom I knew well already, and Jan, whom I'd met only recently, asking them about their impressions of what was going on in the group. Both agreed that the cast wasn't getting the seriousness of their medical situations. It was helpful for me to hear them say that it was important to get the facts out into the open. They agreed that I should be blunt.

My sense of righteousness abandoned me when the moment came. Suddenly, sitting there in that circle of women, I felt like a dark, maybe evil, force—that I was about to block out the sun, take away their hope. Mine would be the unwelcome male voice of reason and science—oh, shit!

I turned to Jan and Mary Sue, needing their reassurance. "Is it ok to do this?" They nodded. Then I took a deep breath and said what needed to be said, wielding my words like violent weapons. "Fifty percent of people diagnosed with metastatic disease die within two years. Eighty-five to ninety percent die within five years."

I couldn't see the blood on the floor, but I knew it was there.

❃

There is a hush, a quiet gasp. Several people appear stunned, taken aback; others are nodding, saddened. The numbers echo around the room. People glance at Mary Sue and Jan, and quickly look away.

Someone breaks the tension. "So this is what hasn't been said." She speaks slowly, looking at Ross, then at the two women with metastatic disease.

"I think we tried," says Mary Sue. "There's a . . . resistance."

"Have the doctors given you a time limit?" the woman asks. "No," says Mary Sue. "They've given me options for treatment."

"A specific prognosis would be hard to take," someone else cautions. "It depends how you take it," replies Mary Sue, describing a friend who, given a 75 percent chance of dying, chose to celebrate her 25 percent chance of living.

"Yes, yes," the woman agrees. "That's a positive attitude."

"A positive attitude is not a cure," someone shoots back.

"I don't want anyone telling me that positive thinking makes a difference," says Mary Sue emphatically.

The conversation circles around the room. Patricia tells us that she has lived for eleven years with breast cancer, not knowing much about metastatic disease at all. "Have I buried my head? A lot of this is very new."

"Everyone is going through their private hell," responds Vrenia. "It's part of the process."

A woman from Act II Studio brings us back to the theater. "It seems to me that we start the drama with Death in the room—the figure of Death, you know, with the black hood and cloak, the scythe."

People are silent. She continues. "Maybe the figure should be in every scene, in the background at least. We know it's there. What we don't know is how people will respond."

Researcher Rant: February 1998: Ross

There was a time, earlier in this century, when the response of family and friends to an individual's diagnosis of cancer was predictably fatalistic. After all, most people died. It was just a matter of time. The word cancer was often left unsaid; it was private, sometimes secret. And physicians and other health care workers conspired with patients to minimize distress by withholding information and limiting discussion. Cancer was not something you talked about.

Times have changed. Cancer, especially breast cancer, now parades across the social landscape of North America. Media personalities cover annual cancer survivorship days, interview famous people who are surviving cancer, and document the efforts of cancer survivors who race dragon boats, climb mountains, and win Olympic medals. Bookstores are overflowing with inspiring stories about personal courage and transcendence in the face of cancer.

The "new glib perception of cheerful survivorship," while preferable in many ways to the "former grim inevitability" (Mayer 1998, 3), poses problems for a sizeable proportion of patients, but especially for those who face advanced disease and likely death. People with advanced disease have to deal not only with the crushing physical and emotional demands of bodily deterioration but must also navigate a course through a societal context that makes little or no room for their circumstances. The experience of losing a breast, for instance—generally not a primary emotional focus for women with metastatic disease—is often central to popular discussions. As in our early meetings, the harsher realities surrounding metastatic breast cancer are unacknowledged, covered up, or resisted. There seems to be virtually no way of talking about cancer other than in the language of survivorship.

Death, then, is not part of cancer's new image. While seriously ill women may sometimes find this reassuring, at other times they can find themselves alienated and misunderstood by those around them (Mathews, Lannin, and Mitchell 1994).

❋

"We had finally addressed 'the D word,' which was death," said Vrenia, recalling the meeting at which Ross read the statistics. "That seemed to be what the project was about at that point, about helping women on their journey to death."

People's fears—about death, about cancer, about the project—bubbled to the surface in interviews after that meeting. "The first transcripts scared the hell out of me," one actor acknowledged. "I wasn't sure I wanted to know more." Breast cancer was imaged as a threat immanent in women's bodies. "When you're dealing with breast cancer there is a real sense of, 'I have two of those, I could be next.'" More than one "well" woman speculated that her involvement in the project tempted fate: "Am I exposing myself to the gods?" A few people withdrew from the meetings, expressing feelings of being overwhelmed.

In thinking back over the first meetings, it was the group's reluctance to take in the difficult truths of advanced breast cancer that remained with Mary Sue. Yet rather than seeing resistance as an obstacle, she affirmed its value. "It was uncomfortable for people learning about metastatic disease in the beginning, and resistance to that, but you know what? There is resistance to hearing it when it's happening to you, so maybe that's what people needed to feel too."

In the course of that meeting, Mary Sue had made reference to the resistance she witnessed in people. "How?" Vrenia had wanted to know. "How have you seen resistance?"

"Well, it's like—Peter and I were driving once, on the highway, and I told him that my oncologist said that a patient of hers with metastatic breast cancer had lived for 23 years . . . "

The story Mary Sue told at that meeting eventually became part of the *Handle with Care?* script. As she pointed out, the group's difficulty in acknowledging the seriousness of metastatic disease parallels the responses of many family members and friends. Women in the focus groups talked about this as well. Even when everyone was aware of the "facts" provided by oncologists, family members sometimes refused to accept, and often refused to voice, the troubling realities that come with a diagnosis of metastatic breast cancer.

"Mary Sue's Rant," from the *Handle with Care?* Script

Not long after my diagnosis, a radiation oncologist told me her longest surviving patient with metastatic disease lived for 23 years. And there it was—long distance hope. I was thrilled. I told my husband on the drive home. "Twenty-three years," I said. "Can you believe it?" "Of course," he replied with that know-it-all look. Well, I lost it. I wanted to pull the car over and whack him one. I was livid because he was dismissing my reality, my fear, my agony. Sure—one patient lives 23 years, and maybe I will too. The fact that one did opens up a world of possibilities. But it's a long shot and it's the not knowing, and being too aware of statistics that makes this disease hell. And I've learned to live with this hell and even become brilliant at it at times—and I don't want him to minimize all that with his glib "of course." When someone says to me, "You're going to live to be a hundred"—that shuts me up. It denies the reality I'm facing. But when someone says, "I hope you live to be a hundred," I can share in that and say, "I hope so too."

CHAPTER FOUR

THEY HAD TO CRY

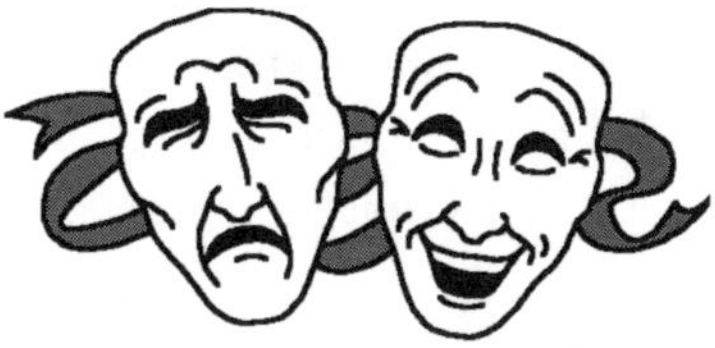

Jan calls Christina at work. "I have this idea for a scene," she says. Christina listens as Jan describes her plans to recreate, in dramatic form, the moment she knew her disease had metastasized. They talk about what Jan is trying to get across, how she thinks it might be staged.

"I wasn't even sure if it needed to be in the show," she recalled later. "But I thought the cast needed to go through it, to hear what it was like, to feel what it was like. We were still having trouble at that point with getting the cast to really understand, and that's what made me think, 'They've got to go through it, they've got to cry.'

"And I also thought, in terms of the progression of the show, if you don't know where she's come from, how can you get her to where she is going?"

And so, at a meeting in March, Jan told the story.

"When the phone rang it was my doctor; I recognized his voice right away. He said, 'I'm calling about your CAT scan. It's an abnormal result.' 'What does that mean?' I said. And that's all I remember saying. I know that he talked quite a bit, 'You need to come in, we need to talk, I think we need to send you back up to Sudbury . . . ' I don't know. I mean, I know he said all those things, because he said them again the next morning, but I really don't remember. Other than I could hear the concern in his voice, and the occasional 'Damn, I'm really sorry. Damn it all anyway, this wasn't supposed to happen,' you know, those kinds of things.

"And I held it all together while I was on the phone. And then as I hung up I kind of fell against the wall and slid to the floor. And this sound came out of me, a sound I'd never heard before, a moan, a wail, this really primal noise. Nadine came flying from wherever she was. She knew it was bad news, she didn't know what level bad news. And I don't think I really understood at that point that . . . that it wasn't curable. I just didn't know what it meant, and I was upset about that.

"Nadine came in and put her arms around me. And the next thing I remember is we were sitting on the kitchen floor leaning against the fridge and sobbing our hearts out. I kept saying to her, 'I'm sorry, I'm so sorry.' Holding my daughter and saying, 'I'm so sorry.'"

Jan pauses. Everyone is transfixed. Then she tells us about the scene she has imagined. She envisions building the tension of it with movement, perhaps with a person in each corner of the stage, crouched over, turning faster and faster. And an absolute bombardment of thoughts: voices whispering, perhaps, and then yelling, the woman's future crashing around her. Voices insisting that the patient breathe, that she pay attention, that she deal with what is happening to her.

Vrenia listens, then stands, and starts to move us into position. We try the scene with figures dispersed across the stage, talking at the patient. It doesn't quite work, Vrenia decides; closer together we generate more energy. She positions one of us directly behind the patient, the other two side by side behind the first. "Stand closer. Shoulders touching. A chorus. Go ahead."

"Don't faint," we say. "Breathe."

"Louder," says Vrenia. "I can't hear you."

"What's the tone?" someone wants to know. "Are we accusing her or begging?"

"Whatever," says Vrenia. "Both."

We try the scene in several ways and eventually the chorus part starts to work. "Don't get into a rhythm," Vrenia instructs. "Listen to one another. Jump in. Scattergun-like."

And then we get stuck. How will the scene end? "With that noise," Jan says. "The noise I made when I found out."

A few people try it, interrupting the "voices" with a cry. It's not right, says Jan. "Anguish. It's about anguish."

"OK," says Vrenia. "You do it."

Jan takes the patient's chair, and the chorus begins. We lean in, trying to push her with our voices, continuing for what seems an eternity. Jan is facing the audience, and beyond her we can see the rest of the troupe watching her face, still, each person tense, wanting it to end.

And then she does it, cries out from that remembered, anguished place.

Almost everyone watching her is teary now, fishing for tissues in purses and bags. And we have learned, in a whole new way, what it means to have metastatic breast cancer.

The epiphany Jan created for the group that day highlights the challenge we faced in relying on the transcripts to allow us entry into the experience of metastatic disease. Everyone involved in the project read at least some of the focus group transcripts. Many people read all of them, diligently underlining provocative quotes, clearly moved by the content. Ann, the research team member who conducted the original focus groups, was able to recall for us something of the tone and nuances of the sessions. The final script of *Handle with Care?* is comprised in no small part of dialogue recorded during the focus group meetings. At the same time, surrounded by mountains of transcripts, Vrenia said, "I still had the feeling we were on the outside of the project—all of us were outside, every single one of us. We hadn't really clicked in."

That we all "click in" was a requirement of this project, for the script was to be forged out of our collective engagement and negotiation with the transcripts, the topic, and one another. The form of the script, Vrenia claimed, would emerge from our work as a group. In her opinion, "clicking in" meant grappling emotionally and personally with the reality of metastatic disease and with the reality that Mary Sue and Jan were living with this diagnosis.

"If we leave it on an intellectual level, nothing is going to happen creatively," said Vrenia. "It was absolutely necessary that we all internalize the realities of metastatic disease. And getting the diagrams and getting the lecture and all that, is not internalizing. Internalizing is feeling something deeply in the gut, having to confront one's own fears of getting cancer or facing a terminal illness, having to figure out how to deal with two special people who are in the group, whom we like and don't want to hurt."

In their assessment of what needed to happen for genuine knowledge about the illness to be created, Jan and Vrenia concur with a chorus of feminist and sociological theorists who insist that emotions be taken seriously (Church 1995; Ellis 1991; Jagger 1989; Narayan 1988; Scheman 1995). Collins writes specifically about empathy as a catalyst for understanding (Collins 1990).

Empathy's catalytic properties became abundantly evident as we worked together on *Handle with Care?* Among the themes important to the women who had taken part in the focus groups, "hope" ranked high. One evening, Vrenia combed through the transcripts for references to hope, searching for the words that would capture its shifting meanings for women with metastatic disease.

"I realized that night when I was hashing through it that my hope was totally hinged on a cure for Mary Sue and Jan and everybody else," she said. "And nothing I could do could lead me to accept that they would die of this disease. Suddenly, there had become a very personal relationship and connection where I didn't want the two of them out of the tapestry of my life. But that's also part of the group dynamic, because the group itself has a life and they became a part of that. And suddenly there was this denial, not denial of their experience or what they are going through, but a really strong fervent resistance to death. To their deaths. . . . But with that also a real understanding of some of the anguish and the fear and the hope and the everything that they and their families and friends must go through because at that point I was living it as well, and I know I was not the only one."

Ann also spoke about the connections developing between members of the troupe and the two women with metastatic disease, and what those connections meant for the project.

"Because Mary Sue and Jan are so totally, marvelously engaging, beyond the usual liking for people, it's almost like falling in love with them in a way, and how vulnerable that makes everyone and the edge it has given things. They have been so much a catalyst. I just don't think it would have been the same at all without them. I don't think that the people from Act II would have had nearly the opportunity to open their hearts. They might have opened their minds and they might have cared deeply about it, but I think Mary Sue and Jan's presence there did an end run."

In Ann's assessment, our "falling in love" with Mary Sue and Jan did not simply enhance other ways of learning about serious illness. Rather, our connection with them "did an end run," evading both an intellectual apprehension of what it means to live with metastatic breast cancer and a (merely) caring engagement with the project.

"They take this role for all of us, the two identified people with metastatic disease who sort of carry our possibilities," said Ann. "It's like an agency for everybody. That vulnerability is an agency, or acts as an agency."

That other kinds of vulnerabilities—life struggles other than cancer—could help us appreciate something of what it is like to be diagnosed with metastatic disease also became increasingly clear as the project progressed. As one woman said, "People began to get the idea that there are related experiences in life that put you into that space where you don't know what is going to happen next and where you are terrified, you don't know what your next move should be . . . things that have happened to you that would make you understand that kind of a space." This realization reflects the assumption that interpersonal interaction can produce understandings that are difficult or impossible to achieve through more unidirectional information giving (Ellis and Berger 2002).

In interviews Christina conducted a few months into the project, several people in the *Handle with Care?* troupe reflected on how their understandings of metastatic breast cancer were changing. A member of Act II Studio credited these shifts in knowledge in part to Vrenia's capacity to speak openly about her own emotional journey, and as well, her commitment to voicing the frightening realities of the illness.

"At the beginning, when we were all feeling our way, Vrenia would introduce what we were talking about, and she kept using the word 'death.' And each time she did, I thought, 'Oh my God.' But I knew it was essential. There was no subterfuge. No euphemisms. Vrenia doesn't 'make nice.' And I think that opened something, because there could be nothing hidden—it was all there, and we had to deal with it."

Researcher Rant: August 2000: Ross

In the early days of the *Handle with Care?* script development, I was unsure of my role in the process, and unclear about how much my presence was required. I hadn't understood how much time would be involved, and was thus only able to attend about half of the meetings. I missed some of the important group-building moments. And I wasn't emotionally affected by learning about metastatic disease in the way that other group members were. Partly, I was very familiar with the issues, having spent more than a decade doing psychotherapy with people with cancer. I'd suffered plenty already through that work and didn't feel the need to induce more in order to be part of this project. But I was also unsettled about my researcher role—whether it kept me separate from what others were experiencing, and, if so, how.

All of this changed as we continued to work together, and as I abandoned my "consultant" approach in favor of that of group member and actor. In an interview with Christina, about six months into *Handle with Care?* I said, "This project is marinated in suffering. Most people tend to have this dichotomy between suffering and, say, hope—or something else. And they see suffering as really awful or horrible. But in one sense, it's all suffering. Every time we do the scene where Jan breaks down, we run into loss and the inevitability of grief, right? And there it is again. But there's something about letting it be there, and not trying to change it or get away from it, that's really very liberating. I think part of what the play does, and part of what we manage to do as a group, is to allow necessary suffering, to make space for it, and to recognize its face appearing all the time."

I was speaking about what is required of all those involved with this project—namely to open themselves to suffering. But I became personally implicated, in ways more direct and profound than have been typical in my research activities. I am not sorry about that; it felt good, in fact.

And, like the rest of our dramatic group, I was now caught between trying to acknowledge the current suffering and wanting to hold off the future. I wanted Jan and Mary Sue to live forever, to defy the bleak odds. Some days I was constantly aware of the river of grief flowing towards us.

I recognize that these experiences of suffering I am describing for myself are not unique to research-based theater or to this particular topic. There are many contexts within which today's qualitative researchers are deliberately opening themselves emotionally to their work (Church 1995; Ellis 1991). Ruth Behar's words are particularly evocative in this regard, "Anthropology that doesn't break your heart just isn't worth doing anymore" (Behar 1996, 177). Drama is one potent vehicle for opening our hearts to the people with whom we work.

I'm partly uncomfortable with what I've just written. After all, whatever emotional challenges I might face with this work are hardly worth mentioning next to the challenges faced by women and men with cancer. I mean, let's not get carried away with this suffering researcher shtick. So I'm looking for a balance here, one that acknowledges my own humanity and vulnerability as researcher, with all of this illness stuff, but also does not let me forget that I am relatively healthy, more privileged, in yet one more way, from most others involved with these projects.

❋

The diagnosis scene as it finally emerged in the script is set in an oncologist's office. The patient is facing the physician, awaiting the results of a bone scan. Three women are standing behind her, heads bowed. The physician says, "I'm afraid the news isn't good" and the patient gasps, turns away; the figures behind her startle upright. As the physician continues to speak, the three figures become her cacophony of thoughts, the personal and cultural voices that define the experience of metastatic breast cancer. The physician forges on with treatment plans, and the chorus intensifies—planning her funeral, anxious for her husband, lamenting her unwritten book—eventually drowning out the physician's voice entirely. Then the chorus pauses; their words trail off, and they lean in. "Breathe," each says, insistently, pleadingly. "Don't faint!"

"Diagnosis" from the *Handle with Care?* Script

(DOCTOR [E], PATIENT [A] & CHORUS [BDC])

E: Good morning, Mrs. Martineau. I have the results of your tests and I'm afraid the news isn't good.

(PATIENT & CHORUS LOOK UP AND TAKE QUICK BREATH IN)

E: We now know that the hot spots that showed up on the bone scan are metastatic lesions.

BDC: I don't want to be here. [LOOK AWAY]

E: I think we should go ahead and start you on treatment and see how things progress. I need to tell you that when breast cancer spreads to the bone, it is no longer curable . . .

D: [FACE FRONT] Oh, no.

B: [FACE FRONT] I'm dying!

C: [FACE FRONT] My kids!

E: . . . but there are treatments that we can give you.

BDC: How's Joe going to cope?

E: Many women do well for a long time, many years in fact.

BDC: [TO DOCTOR] How long do I have?

E: The usual course of treatment is to begin hormone therapy.

BDC: There's so much I haven't done.

D: [FACE FRONT] Hawaii.

B: [FACE FRONT] My book.

C: [FACE FRONT] The garden.

E: So I would recommend that we start you on tamoxifen . . .

BDC: Who's going to look after Mum?

E: . . . which is an anti-estrogen hormone that comes in a pill form.

BDC: Maybe they're wrong.

E: It's effective for many women. And if it stops working . . .

BDC: [TURN AWAY AND PROTECT SELF] I can't cope with this.

E: . . . there are other hormone therapies . . .

D: [FACE FRONT] Update my will . . .

E: . . . and chemotherapy available . . .

B: [FACE FRONT] Music at my funeral . . .

E: . . . and sometimes radiation treatment is used.

C: [FACE FRONT] I'm going to die . . .

D: My kids.

B: Joe.

C: Pain.

E: There may also be some new clinical (B SAYS "BREATHE") trials available here that we might consider. So down the road (B: "BREATHE") we may want to discuss that in more detail.

D: (JOINS B BUT NOT IN UNISON) Don't faint. Breathe . . . etc.

E: The important thing for you to know is that although your cancer has spread . . .

BDC: Breathe, don't faint! (KEEP DOING INTERMITTENTLY, BUILDING THROUGHOUT DOCTOR'S SPEECH)

E: . . . there are things we can do to keep the disease from progressing. And we'll also deal with any symptoms that might occur. Our focus is to provide you with the best quality of life as possible.

(PATIENT COLLAPSES—WAIL. CHORUS BECOMES SILENT)

E: Now I realize this must be difficult for you and I'm going to ask my nurse to come in and spend a few minutes with you. I'm sure you'll have lot of questions later. Do you have any questions now?

BDC: Pull yourself together!

A: [TO DOCTOR] No.

As we worked on the diagnosis scene, our meetings resonated with the seriousness and anguish of metastatic disease. Jan's story, and our translation of it into a dramatic arrangement, evoked the cascade of losses triggered by the diagnosis. The statistics told us that advanced breast cancer—while treatable—was incurable, and often relentless. Once Ross had read the mortality data, one actor said, "Death stalked the room." Women with metastatic disease seemed helpless, their days measured out. The group felt divided between those who were alive and well and likely to stay so for a goodly time, and those who were doomed.

And yet, and yet . . . something else was going on.

Memorybank Drama: April 1998: Christina

We are talking again about the diagnosis scene. Something about it isn't quite right. It has to convey a certain thing, and that thing is anguish. We have to create a scene that accounts for and captures the anguish that women feel at that moment, and we are not there yet.

Jan tries to articulate more of what it was like for her when her doctor told her that her disease had spread. We listen in silence. We are serious, intent. We all want to understand, to feel the proper weight of it.

Someone leans towards Jan, touches her hand. "How did you get from there—from that wail, that anguish—to here?" she asks gently.

"Chinese food," says Jan immediately. "And beer."

"Martinis," Mary Sue chimes in.

For a split second, there is no sound, and then we all erupt. Our laughter is edgy with relief. But it is not only relief. Jan and Mary Sue have broken something, opened something up.

We are supposed to be solemn. The statistics, the patients attached to those statistics, do not admit frivolity. But here they are, laughing with us, urging us on. If Death is in the room, I thought, even she must be smiling.

❋

All of our ideas about what it means to be diagnosed with metastatic breast cancer were constantly tested against the transcripts, against the voices of the women who took part in the original research. They were also, and more immediately, tested against Mary Sue and Jan, against what they said, how they acted, against what they wanted the drama to do and be.

Jan was convinced the group had to get beyond statistics. The project would not move forward, she said, if we were ruled by the image of Death stalking the room. "When the statistics were given out—you know, 85 percent of women with metastatic disease will not survive five years, but 15 percent will (I prefer it that way)—there was sort of hush over the group for just a second. I kind of looked around and I thought, 'Okay, we've said it, now let's pass it, because it can't be what governs us. They have to understand that and know how serious it is, but it can't stop what we're doing.'"

And what we were doing, all of a sudden, was laughing with the two of them. Mary Sue and Jan pushed the medical conversation about advanced disease to the limits of its plausibility. They made it seem unlikely, incomplete. Certainly we had no doubt that they both experienced that anguish, that helplessness. We felt it too, now, in a different way. Yet as often as not, what they said and did—what we said and did together—contradicted the despairing patient invoked by a medical discourse about metastatic disease.

In this way, in how the two of them were living metastatic breast cancer, they referred to and made available to all of us much more complicated sets of realities about the illness. We came to hold, and use, and mix together, what might be thought of as competing ideas: the idea of women with metastatic disease as suffering, and also as impudent, funny, vital, alive.

CHAPTER FIVE
SCRIPTING

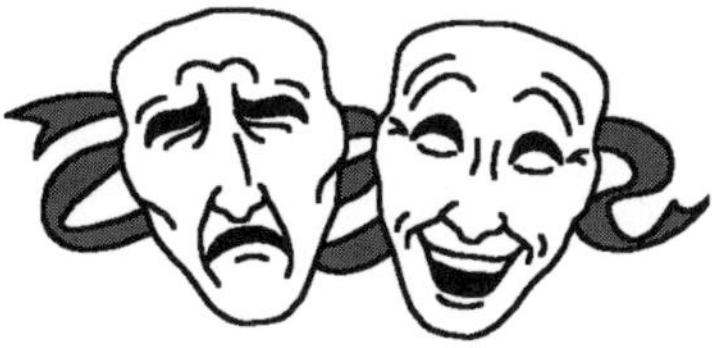

"The word is 'information,'" announces Vrenia. "I want you to do something with this word, in theatrical form." We glance at one another, shuffle a bit. Then we obediently disperse, dragging our chairs into groups of four or five, talking quietly about our task. "On your feet!" Vrenia exclaims. "Get the energy going!"

We stand up, laughing, push the chairs away. Our small group faces one another. Elaine waves a few of the transcripts around. "There's the sense in here of people being overwhelmed with information. It's really coming at them," she says.

"I know this one man, he said when he was diagnosed it was like a truck backed up in his driveway and dumped all this stuff out," says Patricia.

"In the transcripts, women also talk about different kinds of information," says Ross. "Some of it is terrifying, really in your face. Then some of it is more clinical."

"And there's the information that's kind of seductive, that holds out a promise of some sort," Elaine muses.

Jan nods. "People are always calling me when they see something in the newspaper," she says. "You want to tell them to stop, but what if one of them has something?"

"That's the hook," says Ann. "What if one of them has something?" Concurring noises all round.

"So how would we do this, then?" Christina asks. "How would we organize a scene around this?" We pause, trying to imagine it.

"Well, you be the woman," Elaine says to Christina. "Then we could circle around you with all the different kinds of information. I can be the seductive information." Elaine smiles, bats her eyes at us.

"I'll be the clinical kind, walking like this," says Patricia. She grabs a clipboard, holds it in front of her, and furrows her brow, stomping rigidly forward.

"So that leaves me being big and scary," Ross protests.

"You're the man," Patricia laughs.

"Exactly," he says.

"OK, I'll be scary," says Elaine. "You be seductive."

"What should we say, though?" Patricia asks. "Should we just make it up?"

"Why don't we just say the word, 'information,' in all those different ways?" Ross suggests.

We try it out. Three figures swarm around Christina. "Information!" Elaine is commanding, aggressive. Her face practically touches Christina's and she backs off, startled. Ross's seductive information swirls by. It feels cloying, untrustworthy. Christina reaches for Patricia marching across in front of her, the patient trying to grasp the clinical information, slow it down.

"What if one of them has something?" Christina asks plaintively, as Patricia bumps into Ross and starts to giggle.

"It works," says Ann as we gather ourselves back together. "It definitely works."

We perform it for the whole group. Vrenia claps, delighted. But she also wants specifics. "What kind of information? What exactly are people told?"

"Shark cartilage—that's in the transcripts," says one woman. "Green tea."

"People are also told that the conventional stuff is bad for them—like that chemotherapy is bad for you," says one woman. "Or that the jury is out on some drug, or that it's not nearly as good as they thought it was."

We turn to watch a scene that another group has created. A woman—the patient, it becomes clear—is sitting in her backyard with a drink. A series of neighbors appear.

"Just thought I'd come to say hello," says one. "There's no alcohol in that drink, is there?"

"I wish," the woman replies under her breath.

"You shouldn't have the sun in your face," cautions another severely. "Here, let me give you this umbrella."

Another neighbor chirps by. "Are you eating well? Are you getting enough sleep?"

Vrenia is writing furiously, taking it all down.

"There are so many 'shoulds,'" someone says, reflecting on the improvisation. "You should do this—see a naturopath. You should avoid this—no alcohol, no sun."

"You should be upbeat," someone in the group chimes in. "You should have a good attitude."

"But you make it sound like it's all bad," another protests. "Some of it makes sense. And people *are* trying to help."

"Yes, of course. And we all struggle with how to help," says Ann. "But for the patient, it's an effort to sort it out. Moving towards some kinds of information, moving away from others. What others want for you, what you want for yourself. It's a dance, really."

"That's it!" In a second, Vrenia is out of her chair. "A tango—an information tango." She moves around the circle, visualizing it. "Ross, I need you here. Patricia, you come along here. Now, Ross, move towards Patricia with your information, and grab her in the tango hold—like this."

Ross makes a production of it, crouching low to meet Patricia at eye level, sweeping her along. "Try Essiac!" he exclaims. We all chuckle.

"OK, now Elaine, do the same, coming from the other direction," instructs Vrenia.

"Chocolate is very bad for you," Elaine admonishes, carefully moving Patricia across the floor.

"I can't see your faces," says Vrenia. "Skip the tango hold. Try just approaching, and you back up, Patricia. Don't actually touch one another."

We work on it for several minutes, experimenting with the arrangement of bodies. Jan moves into the patient role, trying to react as she might if someone were actually berating her for eating meat or insisting that she take part in a clinical trial. With more confidence, we get faster.

"It's getting overwhelming," says Jan. "I can feel myself getting anxious as everyone comes at me."

"Excellent," says Vrenia.

Meetings went by and we continued to work in this fashion, improvising around themes identified in the original research. Some improvisations were language based; others were entirely silent. Over and over, we took in the written and spoken material and created visual images.

Eventually, we had accumulated a plethora of images, scenes, and quotes, drawn from the improvisation exercises, from our own stories, and from the focus group transcripts.

Yet while many of these "bits" were interesting and evocative, it wasn't at all clear how—or if—they held together. And our meetings didn't seem to be getting us any closer to integrating them. We continued to talk, and to generate images and scenes. June appeared on the horizon, with our promised summer break. No script materialized and the route we would take to produce one remained a mystery.

It was around this time that Ann said, with laughter but not without some urgency, "I would like to see an abstract and an outline."

Memorybank Drama—plus transcript: April 1998: Christina

I am in my kitchen, tape recorder wires trailing around me, microphone clutched to the receiver. I am interviewing Vrenia about the process so far.

Or that's what I appear to be doing. Really Vrenia is speaking a particularly complicated foreign language and I am having trouble keeping up.

Vrenia speaks incredibly quickly: transcripts of interviews with her go on for pages and pages. I am dazzled by her talk. Her voice moves up and down a register; her sentences end with that womanly upward lilt, each statement a half-question. At the same time, she seems utterly, perfectly confident about everything she says.

We start by talking about her worry that the drama won't come together, and her sense that everyone is looking to her to give a structure to it.

Vrenia: I mean the problem is a conundrum. We feel insecure so we look for a form—for answers—to make us feel safe. But safety is not conducive to the search for difficult truths. Risk is essential. But with risk comes fear. Fear is a great spur to creativity but it's uncomfortable to stay with, so we seek safety. I don't know if this is making any sense. It has to do with the creative process.

Christina: Yes, and closing things down too quickly. Or closing down possibilities too quickly.

Vrenia: Yes, exactly. The other thing—I really strongly believe that what happens is, we're going to have another really really difficult period, probably once we start working more intensively, where a huge panic is going to set in, and it's out of that, suddenly, that a crystalline vision will appear.

Christina: Do you have a sense of what the panic will be about? (*Thinking—crystalline vision? Huh? Panic—now* that *I understand.*)

Vrenia: Yeah. People are going to go, "Oh my God, we've got all this material, so much material!" and "We've got all these improvs!" and "Oh my God, what are we going to do? Where are we going to go with this? We've got the show coming up!" Mind you, it won't be quite that panicky because it's really October that we've got the first performance scheduled. I hope we really do feel that the show is looming. Maybe we'll have to invite people to see a preview of it and give ourselves a false performance date, July or something, so it forces our hand. My experience of the nature of creativity is that it's when you've got your back pushed against the wall that you finally cut to the core of the matter and it's likely to come out clearer and stronger than working from a more intellectual, structured approach.

Christina: Yeah. (*Thinking, sounds painful.*)

Vrenia: I really like working on the edge. I've always found in the long run it's best. If you keep exploring at a profound level, focused creativity will blossom literally overnight and it tends to overtake the whole group simultaneously. Suddenly, a current of creative energy takes hold of everyone—it's a creative fever. Things begin to happen with great momentum. Deep truths emerge. It's risky though. [Laughs]. That's the way it's happened before, but what if it doesn't this time? (*Yeah, I think. What if?!*) There aren't guarantees. There's a great temptation to circumvent the process. You need nerves of steel. There are times you feel you're not getting anywhere. You may feel like you're drowning. You may be tempted to grab onto a life preserver. But if you can keep swimming just a bit further, you might discover a wonderful island in that ocean. For the people who are more product than process oriented, it can be incredibly frustrating doing all that swimming around.

I am both drawn and resistant to what she is describing. Where would you put me, I think, process or product? Where would I put myself? I think of myself as process oriented, but there's something about the process here that escapes me. It's not just last-minute-deadline-inspires-brilliance stuff. There's more, something I just can't get a grip on—I feel like I'm sliding around, missing the essential features of it.

Later, I think it is the contradiction between how she speaks, and what she speaks of, that sets me off balance. She has such clarity about the fogginess of it. Such certainty about its unpredictability.

I try to establish some logic.

Christina: And for you, because you've seen it work, your goal is to try and hold off that piece. Hold off the product-oriented types. Calm them down for a while.

Vrenia: Well, not so much calm them down. No, actually, the fear—don't tell anybody this—the panic and fear arising from not feeling secure that there's a product looming is really important. It keeps the search hot. I do think it's part of the process. You know. [Laughs]

Christina: Yep. (*Thinking, nope, I really haven't a clue.*)

❃

The virtues of panic were a theme for Vrenia throughout the creation of *Handle with Care?* Before this interview with her, Ross, Marg, and Christina had discussed the improvisation process she was taking us through.

"It partly makes me crazy and partly I'm just delighted by it," said Ross. "I remember talking to Vrenia on the phone recently, at a time when I was feeling pretty anxious. I was saying to her, 'I can't see how this is coming together, it's just all over the place.' And she's saying to me that in her experience there's no way to get around the fact, you have to come to this place of absolute panic and that she'd tried to avoid it but that's just the way it is."

He pauses, looks up. "And she thinks we're almost there."

Everyone laughs. "Maybe she can tell me when we're there, so I can be absent for that meeting," Christina says, only half-joking.

"I was going to tell her, I think we're there. At least I am." Ross sighs. "I was thinking the other night that I'm never going to do this again, ever. I mean this is a lot harder than writing a paper, as an information dissemination strategy."

"And writing a paper you've had lots of experience with," Marg interjects. "You know the process, and where the points are going to be where you think, 'This isn't a good idea' or 'I've had enough, I can't do anything more.'"

Marg turns to Christina. "I've facilitated educational groups, where you're trying to change perceptions and so on. Those I could understand and know when we're getting to the point of angst. But I've had experience there. I haven't had experience with the theater process."

She looks back at Ross. "I feel like the process we're in right now is so new to me, there are no landmarks, no reference points, so I don't know where I am. Or what's next. Whether what we're going through is normal or not."

Memorybank Drama—plus transcript—resumed: April 1998: Christina

Vrenia: The thing I feel pressured by is that we have a grant and nontheatrical people involved who I don't want to displease. I don't want to alienate them. My own insecurities might make me bolt for safety. Frankly, I could write the script today and hit all of Ross's points from the research. But it would be banal. I sense the heartbeat of something else but it needs time and patience to be heard properly. Whether I can deal with the panic of the research team, I don't know. It depends on how much I can convince them to buy into the process. Right now, I do feel there are several people sitting outside of it.

Christina: That's interesting. And your sense is that the sitting outside of it is . . .

Vrenia: It's a judgmental thing.

Christina: Okay. It's an absence of buying into the process? (*Thinking, are we being judgmental? Maybe we are.*)

Vrenia: Yeah, that's what it is, it's an absence of buying into the process and permitting oneself to join in floundering together. Because I think there's as much floundering on the other side as there is on our side. I mean they are the repositories of the answers but they're no more aware of what's going to happen than we are, and I think there is a desire to get some sort of committed direction. The direction is starting but—do you know what I mean? I don't know how to express this.

Christina: Absolutely. No, you're making perfect sense to me. (*Thinking, we are floundering. We are definitely floundering. And I for one desire direction.*)

Vrenia: And there's almost a wait and see kind of a feeling. [Pause] Now gradually we'll pull people into the circle. . . . Because ultimately it's intoxicating and you can't really avoid it. And in a way, you know, resistance can be really exciting too, because it creates crisis and that's always good.

*

In the early days of creating *Handle with Care?* the research team speculated that some of the tensions surfacing in the project might be "cultural." Our particular research "culture" held, for instance, that knowledge was generated in certain ways. To reach understanding about an issue we observe things, read, search out data, make charts. The "culture" that we were encountering clearly operated in a different way.

In making a case for emotional sociology, Carolyn Ellis argues that "the visualist bias inherent in empiricist social science—that knowledge is seeing—provokes a spectator theory of knowledge" (Ellis 1991, 137). Feminists are among those who challenge the philosophical premise of "observer" knowledge. Traditional knowledge-generating processes are mostly "about" separateness and disinterest; feminist epistemologists, developing alternative theories about how understanding is achieved, propose "connectedness" as an appropriate and necessary standard. In this framework, personal experience is a legitimate basis for knowledge claims; and dialogue, engagement (emotional and embodied), and caring emerge as vital knowledge-creating practices.

In feminist epistemologies, spectator theories of knowledge are often unseated by a commitment to dialogue. The call-and-response discourse mode that Patricia Hill Collins describes occurring in some African American communities discourages—even disparages—"spectators": "For ideas to be tested and validated, everyone in the group must participate. To refuse to join in, especially if one really disagrees with what has been said, is seen as 'cheating'" (Collins 1990, 213).

These ideas, about the obligations members of a community have to the process of generating knowledge, can shed light on how *Handle with Care?* unfolded. When the research team entered the project, we approached group discussions in a manner we deemed respectful. Attuned to our privilege, we took care not to overpower others. We hung back.

It was not until much later, in interviews with participants, that we understood how our "respectful" posture was received. Members of the research team were seen by some as aloof and, as Vrenia said, judgmental. Vrenia was not alone in thinking we had not sufficiently bought in to the artistic endeavor and were unwilling to take the leap of faith the project required. Cheating, indeed.

For Ross, becoming an actor in the drama addressed this problem—a problem about which he was not entirely aware when he agreed to play a role. "The acting group was looking for something more than a research consultant," he explained later. "They wanted more engagement. . . . Acting propelled me to that new level of engagement. And it allowed me to see the practiced role of dispassionate researcher as a danger to the creative process" (Gray 2000, 11).

Researcher Rant: August 2000: Ross

I had not intended to act in *Handle with Care?* Practically speaking, I should not have taken it on. I did not have the time. I have no training.

The contrast with the usual role constructed by and for social scientists is striking. We are trained to be observers. Even with all the recent shifting and moving within qualitative methods—the participatory projects, the cocreation of interviews, the inclusion of the researcher's subjectivity—we are still, in large part, observers. We enter into the worlds of our participants carefully, and with much attention to boundary issues. We stay awhile, and then we exit to analyze, interpret, and write. Some of us go back to check that we got it right. While more qualitative researchers are choosing to be engaged and less protected from the vicissitudes of everyday life, many still stay at arm's length from what they study. It is nothing at all like standing in the participant's body, playing his role, speaking his words, putting oneself on the line.

After years of sitting in front of a computer, typing, and countless meetings with colleagues, discussing, there is something liberating about the movement of my body across the stage. It's exhilarating when I stride to the front of the stage and raise my arms to shout my anger at my sick wife who wants me to go talk with a psychologist:

> If she's going to tell me you've got cancer, well I'm sick of people telling me you have cancer. Everybody I run into is telling me you have cancer. WELL, I KNOW YOU HAVE CANCER!
>
> —From the *Handle with Care?* script

I stick my hands into my pockets and, with the greatest pleasure, revert to an almost forgotten teenage self, telling the doctor:

> CANCER SUCKS! Those treatments you've got mom on, I think they're making her worse. She gets so sick. And everyone has to tiptoe around so she can rest. And dad's always on our case now about doing more around the house. I hate coming home and finding her lying on the couch. It pisses me off! I don't want to lose her.
>
> —From the *Handle with Care?* script

And I find new sympathies for my physician colleagues as I step into their shoes:

> We're human too, you know, and after the patient stops progressing and you've gone through this treatment and that, and there's not a lot more . . . many of us feel that I can't really help her anymore as far as treatments go, and they're sort of frightening to face. These ladies will look at you with these eyes and sort of say, "You've got to do something more." And you know there is nothing more you

> can do, not from the treatment, you know. And the way I get around it is by saying, "I really can't do anything for the cancer but I can help you." Now some will be comforted by that, but some will say, "What do you mean, you can't do anything more for my cancer? There's got to be something more you can do," you know. And it becomes like you almost try to avoid the person the next time around because you've already said that you can't do anything for the cancer, yet they're always still looking for something, you know.
>
> —From the *Handle with Care?* script

❋

Becoming actors in the drama propelled us (Ross and Christina) to new—and unfamiliar—levels of engagement. Initially seated in positions of relatively disembodied observation, we now became physically engaged. We took the stage, becoming subject to the gaze (and judgment!) of fellow actors and the artistic director.

As Vrenia prodded and encouraged us through the endless improvisations, the entire group engaged with issues around metastatic breast cancer in new ways—through our bodies. Each of us "became" patients, doctors, and family members, and felt our varying positions of helplessness, awkwardness, or competence shifting and changing according to circumstances.

The use of improvisation exercises is consistent with a growing recognition of the place of the body in constructing knowledge (Conquergood 1991). Jackson, for example, has written about the importance for ethnographers of reestablishing "the intimate connection between our bodily experience in the everyday world and our conceptual life" (Jackson 1989, 18). Improvisations can elicit the kind of "click moments" feminist theorists attribute to the use of specific consciousness-raising techniques like role playing and simulations (Fonow and Cook 1991).

Our embodied engagement with key themes from the focus group analysis generated knowledge in the group about metastatic breast cancer that the research paper and the transcripts could not. At the same time, however, the knowledge created by the research team took on new significance after we had been through the process of improvisation and group interaction. A member of the theater group reread the research paper and found it meaningful in completely new ways. As Ross put it, there was a kind of "freedom in the improvisation and the articulation . . . people trying to articulate the issues for themselves—like doing an improvisation on information needs. And then there is almost more of a place to connect to the research material from." Having engaged personally and with our bodies the project of giving expression to women's struggles with information, we had expanded the terrain of our understanding. Now even the journal text, the more clearly intellectual of the products generated from the focus group transcripts, came alive. Having spoken the women's words and stood in some way in their places, the textual analysis made sense in a different and fuller way.

At the moment Vrenia insisted that we get on our feet and do something dramatic with the word "information," we could never have envisioned the scene that would emerge. Several conversations, various incarnations, and a generous injection of Vrenia's crafting later, it became part of the script.

The scene follows a monologue by a patient reflecting on the responses of family members and friends to her diagnosis. "Friends, well—you lose some," she says, "and that hurts. They can't handle it. They don't know what to say. You learn to keep up a good front—to look strong so they won't get alarmed and shun you. Then there are the friends and acquaintances who stand by you. They try to help. Oh, yes—they've all got solutions for you—desperately trying to keep you alive by giving lots of free advice."

She moves towards a chair, sits down. "You know," she says deliberately, facing the audience, "I must be the only person in the world who doesn't know how to cure cancer!"

At this point, the audience usually laughs and a second character rushes up. Clutching her arm, this friend propels the woman across the stage, talking rapidly and insistently. "You've got to keep your spirits up!" she exclaims. Her voice drops into teacher-mode. "There's this man who cured himself of terminal cancer by changing his diet—whole grains, organic vegetables, no meats. No alcohol, of course."

They reach the edge of the stage, where another friend whirls around. She too delivers her line rapidly, moving assertively forward. "My neighbor swears by Essiac."

The woman backs up, almost stumbling, to the other side of the stage. This pattern continues (the arrows represent the directions we travel in across the stage):

"Patient Overwhelmed by Well-Meaning Friends," from the *Handle with Care?* Script

(FRIENDS D, C, E, and B; PATIENT A)

D: → You've got to keep your spirits up. There's this man who cured himself of terminal cancer by changing his diet—whole grains, organic vegetables, no meats. No alcohol, of course.

C: ← My neighbor swears by Essiac.

E: → Doctors! What do they know? You'll live to be 100.

B: ← That Dr. De Bello sounds like he's got something. → You should ask your doctor about him.

D: (MOVING A BIT DS TOWARD SR & CURVE) Five doses of chemo? My sister's getting seven.

E: (BEHIND & PUSHING A ←)You know, there's a lot of controversy about tamoxifen.

C: → You're looking great. We're all so proud of you.

B: ← Chocolate isn't really good for you, is it?

D: → I was reading an article that said we have the power to cure ourselves. It's all a matter of attitude.

C: ← Don't worry. You'll be fine. You're a survivor.

E: → You're having a martini? Is that wise in your situation?

D: ← Put some make-up on. You'll feel better. (STAY WITH A)

B: → (PULLING A AROUND) Are you getting enough sleep? (STAY WITH A, MOVE BKWRD)

D: ← (PULLING A AROUND & PUSHING A & B) I wouldn't let them give ***me*** chemo. It pollutes your system, you know.

C: → Chinese Food? Instead of ordering in, why don't I steam some veggies?

E: → (THEN CIRCULAR MOVEMENT) I got you this list of clinical trials off the Internet.

B: (CIRCULAR MOVEMENT—OTHER WAY) Do you want the number of my naturopath?

D: (CIRCLE OTHER WAY) A deep cleansing of your organs. That's what you need.

C: (CIRCLE) My aunt was given six weeks to live. She went to Mexico and got Laetrile and lived to be 175.

B: (CIRCLE) I got some books for you at the library—*How Laughter Cured My Cancer*, *How Meditation Cured My Cancer*, *How Sex Cured My Cancer*, and *Cancer Ward* by Solzhenitzen.

(A DOES DOUBLE TAKE)

D: (CROSS FROM SR IN FRONT & X to USL) Remember. . . . A deep cleansing of your organs is what you need.

B: (IN YOUR FACE) Here's some information.

E: (EFFICIENTLY) The information we have is up to date . . .

C: (SEDUCTIVELY) This information looks promising . . .

A: (OTHERS FREEZE WHILE A SPEAKS) What if one of them has something?

B: (IN YOUR FACE) Information!

E: (CLINICAL) Information.

C: (SEDUCTIVELY) Information.

(THREE TYPES OF INFORMATION CIRCLE AROUND PATIENT AND DUMP BOOKS, PAPERS, MAGAZINES, ETC. ON PATIENT)

The "Patient Overwhelmed by Well-Meaning Friends" scene did not, of course, "really" happen to any of the women who took part in the focus groups, nor did it happen to Mary Sue or Jan. In scripting both *Handle with Care?* and *No Big Deal?* we abandoned traditional realist attempts to describe actual events in the lives of our research participants. Instead, following Vrenia's lead, we concerned ourselves with "making dramatic" common aspects of ill peoples' experiences.

Audience members have told us that the "Patient Overwhelmed" scene captures the acute sense of bombardment with information that many ill people experience. Seeing a woman quite literally pushed around arguably provides a more direct pathway to the truth of her experience than a compilation of statements from the transcripts, or a text-based social science analysis, ever could have. "Drama's just more effective than other ways of learning," said one physician. "I would say it's actually more effective than if you just provide the facts to people. Bare facts are very dry; people are not able to absorb it so much. The drama is simpler; it's easier to conjure up what people are going through."

In another scene in *Handle with Care?* Magda the magician appears, promising to cast a spell on the audience. She warns them that when she says the words, "I have metastatic breast cancer" a cloud will descend on them and they will no longer see her. In her place, they will see a mask—the mask of the doomed woman, the invalid, the victim, or the heroine. A series of battle scenes in *No Big Deal?* work in the same symbolic way. Men and women duck and bob to avoid bombs and machine-gun fire. The maps they've been provided for the campaign are useless to show them how to proceed. The losses they experience are greater than they had expected. With these and other sections of the drama, we invoked an evocative epistemology, crafting scenes that would—we hoped—allow viewers to imaginatively feel their way into ill people's experiences (Denzin 1997).

In the way it is presented, the "Patient Overwhelmed by Well-Meaning Friends" scene may also nudge audiences towards a critical perspective on key cultural messages. The plethora of instructions women receive when they are ill is brought center stage and "poked at." The instructions are delivered relentlessly; they contradict one another and are, at times, quite outlandish. The scene reveals the significant demands on patients to think and act in particular ways, and renders these demands unreasonable, even laughable.

It is also quite clear in the scene that the people so earnestly attempting to deliver the patient of her illness are participants in the patient's immediate social world. As family members and friends, we are prodded into seeing ourselves in their every utterance and gesture. One woman who saw the drama explained that "when friends of someone with cancer see this play, they know the other side. A lot of times they go overboard in helping. There's no in-between.

"A lot of education is needed between the person with cancer and friends and coworkers also," she continued. "They need to see what roles they're playing, and the drama shows that. They see it played out. They're going to see themselves."

The actors rushing back and forth across the stage monitor the patient, assess her needs, instruct her in certain choices or behaviors, discipline her if she strays. Once she is constituted as patient, she is "fair game" for surveillance (Morgan 1998, 93). And while surveillance may sound ominous, its key feature is the way it is embraced by the actors in the scene—and each of us in our daily lives—as a moral undertaking (Gastaldo 1997).

Others might suggest that the scene implies a critique of the patient as "consumer." In relation to health and illness, "consumer culture latches onto the prevalent self-preservationist perception of the body, which encourages the individual to adopt instrumental strategies to combat deterioration and decay" (Turner 1992, 165). In this scene, a patient's "empowerment" becomes her capacity to take charge of a vast array of products and strategies for health. The scene turns on a discourse of choice. When choice is constituted in terms of consumerism, everything becomes a product. The patient is told to pick her attitude like she would select an evening meal. Information is the quick fix, the best buy.

The key, of course, is that information, the products and strategies, may well be useless in terms of a woman's survival or her ability to cope with the illness. And as a "consumer" in a constant state of anxiety that one of the "salespeople" might "have something," she may well be distracted from efforts to articulate her deeper, less tangible needs and desires.

Not everyone saw it that way, of course. After our first performance in Toronto for health professionals, Christina returned to her "day job" at a provincial breast cancer organization. Staff from the organization had attended the performance. One of them walked into Christina's office. "As a breast cancer survivor, I felt disempowered," she declared. She went on to say that she felt the drama portrayed women with metastatic breast cancer as powerless, especially in relation to information. She was disturbed by the message oncologists might take from the performance—that women with metastatic disease cannot generally integrate or use information, and thus that health professionals are justified in withholding information, managing it "for" women.

In an interview with Ross, Christina spoke about what it was like to hear that, particularly anticipating the performance scheduled for that evening, when other colleagues would be present. "I remember feeling the weight of the criticism and just trying to protect myself against it. Not really being able to engage with it at the time, but also not wanting to be defensive, so just trying to keep it at some distance."

Later, in a paper for one of her courses, Christina tried to look at the drama from a variety of feminist perspectives, hoping to settle on an analysis that attended to the criticism, and also reflected her own beliefs about health information.

Excerpt from a Paper Written for CHL5109H: Gender and Health, December 1999

Handle with Care? emerged from a study that explored the information needs of women living with metastatic breast cancer. The drama, based on that research, clearly renders information problematic. It surfaces women's difficulty in handling—in understanding, absorbing, and managing—

information. This paper discusses instances in which *Handle with Care?* comments on a physician's role in providing women with information about their illness and its treatment. At different points, the script can be seen to chastise doctors for their failure to offer comprehensible information, to provide them with encouragement and tools to do so, and to let them off the hook completely.

Even more critically, however, the drama questions the value of information to women living with metastatic breast cancer. From many feminist locations, this is an immensely dangerous move. The women's health movement has fought long and hard in this country for women's rights to information about our bodies, our health, the diagnoses we encounter, the treatments medicine offers. To question the value of information—regardless of how we qualify or contextualize or explain our questions—may well collude with the forces that would render us forever and only "patient."

In one scene in the drama, a woman sits facing her physician across his desk. He is talking to her about her disease:

E(DOCTOR): Disease progression, blah, blah, blah, blah, blah. Treatment options blah, blah, blah. Side effects, blah, blah, blah, blah. Prognosis, blah, blah, blah. What would you like to do?

A(PATIENT): I'm not in the medical profession and I found I was given almost too much to decide on my own. And maybe deep down I didn't want that responsibility.

. . .

D, E, C, AND B, ALL DOCTORS, LINE UP ACROSS THE STAGE WITH THEIR BACKS TURNED TO

THE AUDIENCE. THEY ARE SILENT AS A, THE PATIENT, MOVES RAPIDLY BACK AND FORTH BETWEEN THEM AND ACROSS THE STAGE.

A: (TO D) I'm feeling bombarded. (TO E) What would you do if this was your wife? (CROSSING IN FRONT) This is too overwhelming. (TO B) I want more information! (CROSSING BEHIND) I'll think about it tomorrow. (SITTING IN CHAIR) Slow down. Too much, too fast. (JUMPING UP, TO C) Can't you do that for me? (CROSSING OUT FRONT) Give me time to digest this. (TO D) Don't tell me too much. (TO E) I want it straight. I can take it. (CROSSING BEHIND E TO CENTER, HANDS ON EARS) I'm not ready for all this. I'm so sick of all this. I don't want to hear about it anymore!

—From the *Handle with Care?* script

The first moments of this scene are enough to have Illich (1976), and feminists theorists who follow his structuralist critiques, spinning—in their graves and otherwise. Illich's thesis is grounded in individual responsibility. For patients to give up responsibility for their own bodies "is worse than forgoing professional medical treatment" because when specialized knowledge about the patient's body is not available to her or him, "the patient's body becomes separated from the self, with a corresponding loss of human autonomy and dignity" (Bologh 1981, 193). Certainly, the scene highlights just how specialized medical information can be. More problematically, it may also suggest that the effort to understand is utterly futile—how, after all, is one to decipher "blah blah blah"?

At the same time, this scene might be understood to problematize the subjectivity constituted by discourses of informed consent: the autonomous decision maker.

> The paradigm offered for informed consent is built on a model of . . . patients who are accustomed to making decisions about the course of their lives and who possess the resources necessary to allow them a range of options to choose among. Decisions are constructed as a product of objective calculation on the basis of near perfect information. (Sherwin 1998, 24)

As Sherwin points out, most patients do not live in these ideal circumstances. Yet there is little recognition of this truth, and no satisfactory frameworks available for health professionals about how to proceed when responding to patients and situations that do not fit the paradigm.

Feminists writing from Foucauldian locations, and from the structuralist perspective Sherwin employs, might highlight the patient's complaint that she was given almost too much to decide *on her own*. Here, the scene can be read as a critique of contemporary choice-making models that assume individuals can and do make health care decisions in an entirely independent way, detached from the web of relationships in which they live their lives. It could also point to the inadequacy of supportive care resources for patients in this era of cuts to health and social services.

Rather than assessing whether *Handle with Care?* constructs women as able or not to manage breast cancer information, postmodernists would likely applaud the ways the drama portrays a multiplicity of stances in relation to breast cancer information. In some scenes, women clearly want and value information, and manage it adeptly. In others, women struggle with information, and, as in parts of this scene, confirm certain stereotypes of women and patients. In a parallel way, some physicians in the drama speak and act their commitment to patient autonomy; others demonstrate blatant paternalism. These, of course, are the extremes: the strength of the drama, from a postmodern perspective, is in the ways it casts light on the ground in between.

Proponents of this theoretical school would resist making—or "finding" in the drama—any general statements about women, or about patients, or about physicians. Rather, they would emphasize the contingent nature of the patient "selves" foregrounded in *Handle with Care?* and in this scene particularly. The drama highlights the ways women's capacities to manage information are related to circumstance, vary between women, and vary from day to day—sometimes hour to hour—for any one woman. This scene demonstrates the latter point beautifully: the same woman is, in one moment, entirely prepared to manage information, and in the next quite overwhelmed by it; in one instant wanting control and decision-making authority and, in the next, asking others to take it on. In keeping with Denzin's standards for subversive performance texts, the scene resists the notion of a unified subject (Denzin 1997).

In the final scene of the health professional version of *Handle with Care?* the patient and the physician sit facing one another. There is no desk between them. The doctor says, "I'm sorry" and the woman gasps, sinks back in her chair. Three figures start to walk around them:

C: I am chemotherapy, and I have nothing more to offer here.

B: I am your friend and I am so distressed by what is happening to you, I have nothing more to offer here. (COMES TO A STOP BEHIND PATIENT'S CHAIR)

A: I am seven years of training, residency, fellowship, books, research articles, your white coat, and your stethoscope, and I have nothing more to offer here. (COMES TO A STOP BEHIND DOCTOR'S CHAIR)

C: (ENTERING BETWEEN DOCTOR AND PATIENT) I am hope. Is there still room for me here?

D: INTERVIEWER: Doctor, how do you cope, working with very ill patients?

E: DOCTOR: I don't know. Who says I'm coping?

❋

Like the entirety of *Handle with Care?* this scene is open to a wide range of feminist interpretations. Some would use it to critique the drama's collusion with all that would oppress women, all that would dismiss and patronize patients. Others might take the scene as compelling evidence of the drama's emancipatory power. I have aimed in this paper to locate myself in this discussion, so I'll conclude with a script of my own—overdrawn, but there it is, it's drama.

My structuralist feminist self: How utterly pathetic. Leaving women with "hope." We struggle for millennia for the material resources to take charge of our health and they want us to be satisfied with hope. This scene totally buys into the pat-her-on-the-head, feed-her-a-crumb-and-she'll-be-happy routine, the remorseless medical routine that locates and confirms women as powerless, entitled to nothing but platitudes. You think they would offer a man hope? Right. Get a grip.

My postmodern self: Ah, but look at it. All the structures we create to separate them, all the imputed oppositions, are utterly disrupted. They are both abandoned; neither can cope. Vulnerability is the defining characteristic of "patient" and the doctor claims it; it disperses, becomes common between them. This scene directs our attention, in a most liberating way, away from the relentless pursuit of certain kinds of information. It surfaces our profound need for other kinds of knowledge: how to withstand the abandonment of what you have been able to trust, how to live with despair, how to encounter death. The physician's agency as a human being, with a capacity as limited—and as wide—as a patient's, is invoked in this scene. Hope is what matters here: hope for both of them.

My (post) structuralist feminist self: The critical part is action. And not just any action. The question becomes: What action does witnessing the drama allow, make possible, enable? Denzin, in his discussion of critical, poststructural narratives, claims that "ethical talk" (interaction that cherishes justice, and each person's dignity) moves forward because individuals are able to share one another's point of view (Denzin 1997, 277). Certainly this scene, and the drama as a whole, offers the possibility of increased understanding (though not necessarily consensus) between physicians and patients. The test, again, is in the action: if the drama shifts—in the direction of dignity and justice, how a doctor, or a patient, perceives and acts in the world—it has succeeded. Now there's an evaluation study waiting to happen.

❃

At the outset of *Handle with Care?* separateness characterized our meetings. Early interviews describe two "cultures," a research culture and a theater culture. Distinctions between those who had breast cancer and those who did not seemed rigid, unbreachable. The women with metastatic disease seemed "different," as did, in some ways, the women living with a primary breast cancer diagnosis. It was as if the people in the room occupied a series of islands with only the occasional communication from the rest washing up on each shore.

Yet over the course of creating *Handle with Care?* something important changed. Ross put it this way: "These groups—people who are well, and people who had been sick but are now well, and then people who are not well—found their way to some common ground. The shift in tone is, in part, everybody moving into the space occupied by the ill women, and taking that up, being willing to take that up. I thought it was distinct cultures that was the source of most of the fracturing early in the project. But I think over time it is, to me, much more of an existential thing where people have had to make the effort to move themselves in the direction of really confronting mortality and loss. And so there is, in some ways, a sadness underlying everything. But there is also just a real sense in which people are really on board with the experience of women with metastatic disease."

CHAPTER SIX
STEPPING INTO THE SPOTLIGHTS

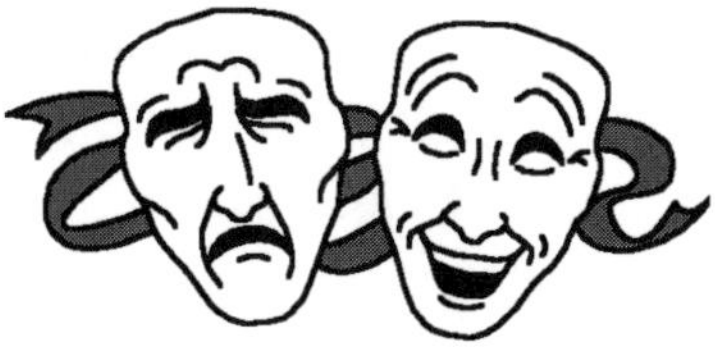

Handle with Care? was, in many ways, an audacious project. Think of it: Oncology Grand Rounds. Surgeons, oncologists, radiologists, gathered together in a lecture hall. White coats, pagers, an hour of immeasurably precious time—for what? For a drama? A *play?*

While the script was still in its early stages, members of the troupe tried to imagine how *Handle with Care?* would be received at regional cancer centers. Hope and worry entered into uneasy equilibrium.

"What happens in theater, when it changes someone?" asked one of the women from Act II Studio. "You get an epiphany. I mean, that's what you're looking for, in my opinion. At the end, there's been a transformation, a transformation in attitude, a transformation in the emotional connection, the way you relate, the way doctors relate.

"Now, I mean, that's not going to—unless you get something wonderful, it's not going to happen, you know."

Vrenia talked about the extraordinary kind of theater this setting demanded. "There will be doctors whose worlds we have to honor, in a way, and be compassionate with, while at the same time hoping to kind of open things up, to create at least an awareness and a sensitivity in some doctors who already feel besieged."

"It has to be clever and it has to be respectful and it has to be tight," said Ann.

"Within the first thirty seconds, most of them, all of them probably, will have twigged to what's going on," Vrenia said. "And we have to grasp them so they don't go 'Oh, God'—because I fully expect that to be the reaction, if what we have is not brilliant. So that's my great fear."

Members of the research team, recalling their own experiences at Grand Rounds, anticipated a less-than-enthusiastic welcome.

"I have presented at Rounds," said Ann in an early interview. "And I can tell you, it's just not a fun group. They are laid back—they are doing you a favor, you know."

"I felt quite scared," Marg said. "Worried about what was going to happen and worried—if we ever did end up with a production—about how it would be received. Thinking about some of the audiences I know at other cancer centers, colleagues, and my perception of how they might react—I could see some getting up and walking out, some making very scathing remarks about the value of doing this. Scathing remarks about how we had it all wrong, that it wasn't like that at all. Just a wall of negativity. You see, I've had that happen to me after presenting material that was outside their comfort zone. The reaction on their part is one of getting defensive, being critical, trying to find the weak points. It's a pattern of behavior within the group."

*

Three cars are moving east along Highway 401 towards Kingston, having left from three different parts of central Ontario. Ross is driving the first car, Elaine and Patricia are with Jan in another, Christina and Ann are in the third. The rain is relentless. Everyone peers ahead, searching for lane markers and road signs. The pavement is awash with water.

When Christina and Ann reach the hotel, Ross has already checked in. We haul our luggage to the desk, find our rooms, gather again in the lobby. Perched in gaudy wingbacks, we wait for Jan, Patricia, and Elaine to arrive.

It is almost thirty minutes later when they pull up, weary and out of sorts. Blocks from the hotel, another driver slid through a red light and hit Jan's car. We exclaim concern, murmur sympathy when we realize they're okay.

Once everyone is more or less settled into the hotel, we pack Ross's car and head for Kingston's teaching hospital. Our plan is to rehearse in the room where we'll perform tomorrow morning. We can't leave the set up, though; another group needs the space before us.

The auditorium is cavernous. A wall of seats rises straight up in front of us. We stand there for a moment, gazing upwards. "Yikes," says Christina.

"Where are you going to look when we're performing?" Patricia asks Jan. "Here, this row," Jan says, making her way up the narrow set of stairs between the seats.

Ann stakes out a place in the front where she will sit to prompt us if we forget a line. We assemble the set, walk through the script. Mostly we remember our parts.

"You'll need to project more," Elaine says to Christina. "It's a big space."

We take the set down again, pack it into the bags, trundle out to the cars. Somewhere we find food, then disperse gratefully to our rooms.

Far too soon, it is morning. Each of us appears purposefully in the lobby, dressed all in black. Ross's sleeves are rolled to his elbows. "Those will have to come down, you know," Jan says.

"I know," mutters Ross.

Once again, we load ourselves and the props into cars and find our way to the hospital. Our footsteps echo through the underground parking lot. Ross and Christina have the heavy bag of props between them. It bangs against the doors as we struggle through the maze of corridors.

In the narrow hallway outside the auditorium, half crouched under a set of stairs, we assemble the set. People in white coats appear and disappear—nurses, residents, a few physicians. Some of them glance curiously at us.

They have no idea that they'll be seeing a drama. Alert to the possibility that oncologists might break their habitual attendance at Rounds if they knew they would not be getting "the usual," Ross has neglected to mention that a drama will take place, and instead booked himself as the guest speaker. As far as everyone here knows, a psychologist from Sunnybrook will deliver a lecture about metastatic breast cancer, at 10 A.M. Probably there will be slides.

As the auditorium door opens and closes, we can hear the low drone of the lecture currently underway. We will have less than five minutes to set up after they leave.

We hang large pieces of paper with quotes from the focus groups on four banners. Jan grips two of the banners tightly, preparing to carry them through the door. Elaine rummages around for clips to secure the box Patricia will emerge from in the first scene. Elaine and Christina will transform the box into a desk for the doctor, once Patricia begins her "perfect patient" monologue.

Christina clutches the drum that will mark the ends of scenes. The sound of this drum resonates for Ross in special ways; it is his, a gift from friends, used in Zen Buddhist chanting. Initially, he was hesitant about having it in the drama. He didn't want to introduce any formal religious symbolism, and he worried that it might be damaged. But one day Elaine talked about the spirit of *Handle with Care?* and Ross decided that the risk of damage was fine to take.

Ann stands by, handing us various bits and pieces, folding the carry bags under the stairs.

There is no room to pace.

Memorybank Drama: October 1998: Christina

I remember distinctly the hum in my head, remember thinking over and over: What on earth am I doing here? This is preposterous, I thought. Clearly, they have the wrong person. I'm the one in the background, prodding things along. The one on the sidelines, cheering. I can do a presentation when I need to—the lectern, the notes. I can do that. But it is simply unfathomable that, moments from now, I am going to stand in front of these people with no more than myself, and some vague memory of words, gestures, positions on a stage. Simply unfathomable.

❃

The auditorium door opens and people filter out. "Ready?" Ross opens the other door, swinging in two of the banners.

We hurry everything into place. Various shaking hands organize the papers, the stethoscopes, the telephone. We take our positions, Jan and Christina on one side of the stage facing Patricia and Elaine on the other, Ross with his back to the audience.

Patricia glances out into the auditorium. People are still coming in, but it seems almost empty; perhaps thirty people dot the expanse of seats. Their faces are quite blank. They seem utterly unmoved by this odd flurry of activity in their space, these five black-clad figures assembled in front of them.

One person is familiar. Mary Stewart, from the local breast cancer group, smiles warmly at us.

A staff person from the cancer center says a few words and turns the floor over to us. Jan looks up at Elaine and Patricia, nods once. It's time.

Jan strides in front of the banners, turns to face the audience. "I was devastated the second time, worst than the first, because it is worse." Her voice is strong and clear. Patricia speaks next, moving in from the other side of the stage. "It's not any easier for a seventy-four-year-old woman to die of breast cancer than it is for a thirty-three-year-old. It's unjust to say that because you're seventy-four you should just grin and bear it."

"I needed to hear and talk to women who were living with metastatic disease," Elaine chimes in, following Patricia towards the center of the stage. It's Christina's turn; she moves forward, speaking as she walks, "I didn't even tell my sisters, I felt so ashamed."

Jan again. "As long as I get up, get dressed, and put on my make-up, everybody thinks, 'Oh, mom's okay. Mom's gonna be fine.'" And then Elaine: "I found I was given almost too much to decide on my own." And Christina again: "Not being able to get behind the fear, that's the biggest enemy."

Jan walks towards the audience, speaking directly to them. "My doctor didn't give me a limited amount of time, but she also said she wasn't God. She also told me she would never give up. She said there's treatment coming out every day and I'll always be there to fight for you and give you hope. . . . I'll never abandon you." Elaine walks forward, her hands outstretched. "You feel like you've got this bomb ready to go off inside you!"

We move into the next scene, then the next.

Memorybank Drama: October 1998: Christina

It seems to be going okay, but I can't quite tell. I can't quite breathe. My heart is pounding so hard my whole body is shaking.

I take my seat in the doctor's chair, and Patricia sits next to the desk. Elaine narrates the scene. "One of our support group members was very ill and her family doctor asked her to ask the oncologist if Taxol was an option. When she did, the oncologist said . . . "

I pick it up, the voice of the doctor: "This is coming from your support group. It's really not helpful. Taxol isn't an option. All you women do is sit around and talk about your medication."

I stand, walk away from my "patient" and towards the health professionals in the audience. "Honestly, it's time consuming," I confide, trying to look at them. "Especially the women who have a lot of information from support groups, you know . . . "

And then I can't remember. I can't remember the next line. My mind grasps for it, stumbles. I can hear myself talking but I know I'm not making sense. Ann is in the front row; I should ask for my cue. I feel like I'm babbling. I have to stop.

Somehow, I muster a tone that conveys "I'm finished now." A second hangs, and then Patricia moves forward. I am flooded with gratitude to hear her voice.

"So what happens," she says, "when you do have information and are asking questions, and you're actually being reprimanded for having too much information? It isn't too much information. I'm only asking, 'What's my next line of defense?' I'm fighting for my life!"

The rest of the performance blurs by, and then, mercifully, we are done.

And—wonder of wonders—they are clapping.

❋

"There was a lot of nervousness among us about how it was going to be received," Patricia recalled later. "I was properly terrified," Elaine confirmed.

"And I think once we had done it," Patricia continued, "there was this real joyful feeling, we all wanted to hug and kiss one another because, boy, we'd got it over with! And then people asking if it could be shown in other medical settings and suddenly you realized that it's not just our little group that's putting something on, it's like people are really interested and really want to take it further."

As the applause ebbs away, Ross heads for the lectern. "We're really pleased to be here," he says. "This is our first performance of *Handle with Care?*" He continues for a while, explaining the origins of the drama and inviting the cast members to introduce themselves.

He rolls up his sleeves. "Now we'd like to hear your responses to the performance," he says to the audience.

A man in the front row—an oncologist, we learn later—speaks first. "You did very well," he says. "I would say it was fairly accurate, from the point of view of the patient and of the doctor. It was unique."

"The voices at the beginning, from the women, that was superbly well done," someone else says.

Another man puts up his hand. "I'm a second year M.D. student, and I learned more in this hour than I could ever have learned from a dozen lectures and textbooks."

"I'm a physician," says another, "and I'm going to be seeing a woman with metastatic breast cancer in an hour. This stuff is really going to stay with me. It's very powerful."

A few people want to know about the focus groups, and about how we chose quotes from the transcripts. Ross handles most of the questions as the rest of us sit, rather stunned, in silence. When we get up to leave, they applaud again.

In the car, we grin at one another in amazement, recalling what various members of the audience said. Each of us recounts to the others the conversations that took place with individual nurses and doctors who had approached us while we packed up the set.

We arrive back at the hotel limp with relief. But it is not over. This evening we are expected at the Kingston Public Library, to perform the community version of *Handle with Care?*

We change into regular clothes and a few of us head out to wander around Kingston, winding up and down the streets, poking through shops. The wiser among us nap at the hotel. In the late afternoon, we reassemble and head for the library.

"You're with the play?" the woman at the desk asks. "How did you guess?" Patricia smiles back, her gesture encompassing our black attire, the bags of props.

The woman directs us to the room, which is large and airy. Watercolors line the walls. The stage, however, is small—smaller than any space we have rehearsed or performed in. We survey it gloomily. "I wonder if we really need the stands for the banners," Christina mutters. She sets to work trying to pin the banners to the back wall so we can have more stage space.

"We'll need to watch the edges there," says Patricia, pointing to the gaps on either side of the stage with a stair to the next level. Later, Jan steps backwards and stumbles down one, jarring her back. We all wince, imagining the pain.

Elaine and Patricia assemble the desk and try to gauge the distance it should be from the back wall and the side of the stage. Too far back and we won't be able to get behind it for the family scene. Too far over and Ross won't be able to get around it when he is the doctor.

Finally, we agree on positions for the set, and mark the stage with tape. It is too late to do a full rehearsal. We decide to run lines. Ross and Christina sit on the stage, the rest bring chairs around to form a circle.

A woman comes in the back of the room; she hovers. Is she part of the breast cancer group? She doesn't approach us. A few other people filter in. They speak with her, turn to look at the walls.

She is here for an art opening, we realize eventually, and she is the featured artist. This is awkward; we are in a space probably quite important to her, and ignoring her work. Ann goes over to speak with her and we lower our voices, huddle together.

Elaine laughs, then stifles herself. "We look like some cult, preparing for a ritual," she says. She looks up at Ann, who has a red jacket over her black outfit. "Ann must be our leader."

We start to giggle. Jan restrains us, trying to get us focused on the lines. We plunge on, feeling the giddiness just below the surface. We haven't eaten much. The morning's adrenaline is wearing thin.

The artist and her entourage disappear into the next room.

We reach the family scene. Ross is the son, exploding with pent-up anger at his mom's illness.

"Cancer sucks!" he says vehemently. "Those treatments and pills you give her—I think they're making her worse. She gets so sick. And then everyone has to tiptoe around so she can rest. And dad's always on our case to do more around the house. And you can never speak your mind because dad gets mad if we upset mom. I hate coming home and seeing her lying on the couch . . . "

These are the lines from the script—what Ross says, though, is "I hate coming home and seeing her lying on the floor . . . "

This is, for no good reason, unbearably funny. We dissolve into laughter, leaning on chairs, wiping tears, gasping for air. It is a huge relief to laugh. At the same time, it makes us uneasy about tonight. Will we hold it together?

We find the washrooms, scrounge for something to eat, return to the room. By this time, people are taking seats and flipping through the program. The women from Breast Cancer Action Kingston welcome us warmly. They want to know how it went at the cancer center and Mary helps tell the story, explaining to us who some of the audience members were.

We are watching the clock. As it moves towards 7:00, we take deep breaths and line ourselves up.

It feels entirely different here, in this space. We are nervous, but not wildly so; and as we move along, we can feel the audience with us. This is new: this is extraordinary. They chuckle at Patricia's "perfect patient." When the diagnosis scene begins, they gasp with us; we can feel them absorbing the anguish of it, taking it in. Later, we hear a few people crying.

We come to the family scene, and the contrast with our raucous rehearsal is stark. We are focused, engaged. Christina looks at Jan. Her longing for Jan to stay well flows into her "daughter" character, mixing with her own fears about illness: "Am I going to get cancer too? I'm afraid to ask her. I want to go away to university next year, but maybe I should wait, maybe I should try and be here for her. I don't want to lose her." Next to Christina, Ross's frustration and grief at his "mom's" illness radiate from his body. Everyone in the audience is still.

We are reaching the end. Jan is preparing herself, mapping out her next moves. She turns from the back and speaks directly to the audience: "Who needs seventy-eight jars of homemade dill pickles?"

People chuckle. "I do!" she exclaims, and sets off toward the front of the stage.

"It's a long story," she admits, "but I've established myself as the best dill pickle maker in my family. It's a title I bear proudly and work hard to maintain. This year, I thought I might have to relinquish my standing 'cause I needed some treatments. And I know from the last ones that I'd feel yucky after. But large egos are hard to stifle and my reputation was at risk. I enlisted the aid of a good friend who volunteered to do the heavy jobs—like wash the cucumbers in my washing machine."

We can feel the audience startle, then laugh. They are completely with her. Their enjoyment of the scene, of Jan, of the nuggets of meaning about illness embedded in the common rituals of laundry and pickles, is delicious to us.

Excerpt from "Pickle Piece" from the *Handle with Care?* Script

Yup—you heard right. Cold water, gentle cycle, one third of a bushel at a time and for heaven's sake, don't spin dry—unless you want relish. So anyway, this friend put the cukes in the machine, swished them around for ten minutes, took them out and hauled them up to me in the kitchen—where I sat like a queen bee stuffing jars with garlic, dill weed, and cukes. When the brine was ready, I'd pour while my friend tightened the lids. Then she hauled them back to the basement to the cold cellar. I thought—a person could get used to such help. I wonder how long she'll let me get away with it?

Patricia moves in, finishes the scene: "Yes, they've told me that it's incurable," she says, her voice heavy, acknowledging the truth of it. "That's a pretty scary word.

"But I prefer to break it down into three parts—IN—yes, I know I'm in for a fight; CURE—I prefer to believe one is just around the corner, and, ABLE—as long as I'm able, I prefer to hang onto the hope for a cure."

The audience is silent. People are nodding, confirming. Ross strides forward from the back. "The hierarchy of hope!"

"I hope they find a cure," says Patricia. Jan walks forward. "I hope they'll keep finding new drugs to treat me with." Elaine moves in from the right, and Christina follows her: "I hope I won't be in pain." "I hope my doctor stays with me until the end."

We take our places across the stage. Eyes in the audience move across us as we each speak. "I hope I live to see my son graduate from high school," says Jan. "I hope people won't forget me," says Patricia. "I hope I'll be able to cope with whatever I have to deal with," Christina says.

Elaine is next. "I hope my husband learns to cook—better than he did last night." Again, people in the audience are smiling. Jan plants her feet, takes a breath: "I hope I live long enough to see this government booted out of office." There is a hoot of astonishment, then they start to clap—loudly. When the applause subsides, Christina speaks again: "I hope my mind stays clear." "I hope I can find shoes to match my dress," says Elaine. "And I hope," says Jan, drawing them along with her, "that the cucumber crop is a good one, next year."

Jan waits a beat, and we turn in ragged unison to face the back with her; we count to three, and Ross leads the turn to face the audience. We step into line, join hands, and bow.

And we hear their hands coming together, again and again and again.

Our memories of that performance are wonderfully sweet. "Perfect strangers coming up and hugging me afterwards," Patricia said. "It kind of took your breath away, you know, you wanted to cry."

"The support group people were very friendly in the beginning, before the show," Elaine recalled. "But I was waiting for that feeling that we were connecting—and I feel that we really did connect. I felt that these people were responding. That was my first experience in that kind of exchange, for people to be sufficiently touched, to come up and speak to us."

"Everybody felt the intensity," said Ann. "It was the moment of truth."

"Ross was beside me when we took our bows," Jan said. "And, when I turned to him, the grin on his face was just so touching, like he knew we'd done it, that the people in the audience loved what they'd seen. He just beamed, you know. And that's a very special memory for me because after we took our bows, I stepped back and turned to him, and he put his hand on my shoulder, and that look on his face was just pure joy."

❋

When our editor, Arthur Bochner, read a draft of this book, he wasn't satisfied with our description of the Kingston performance. "It sounds too much here like your primary goal was to be loved by your audience," he complained. "Sure, you wanted them to appreciate the work you'd done, but this overemphasis on 'the standing ovation' detracts somewhat—or runs the risk of detracting—from the messages." He encouraged us to explore what the audience loved in the drama itself, and describe how else (beyond applause) they responded. "I'd like to see you emphasize some of the other reactions that were evident," he wrote. "Empathy, sorrow, fear, a collective sense of the sadness and possibilities of the human condition."

We could see Art's point, of course, and felt a bit rueful about our self-centered narrative and our narrow construction of audiences. And yet thinking about it more, and remembering back to the time of that performance, it became clearer to us that in the early days we were, in fact, desperate to be loved—or at least not run out of town. Or dismissed. Or berated for an inaccurate/destructive/Pollyanna (pick one or all of the above) representation of women with metastatic disease, or of oncologists. Initially, all we "heard" from audiences was that we had managed to avoid our worst-nightmare scenarios. Ross still seemed to have a job. Chris hadn't been banished from the breast cancer community. And, of course, we had all made it through the performance; despite all our predictions, no one had fainted or fallen over. Yet it was sometimes several minutes into audience questions before we started to breathe normally.

The other reality, as well, is that most people who spoke after performances were unreservedly positive about the drama; it took us a while to find the nuances, to engage more fully in their responses.

Later in this book, we capture more of what went on for people who witnessed *Handle with Care?* and what went on for us when we better understood how they had been affected by it.

For now, though, what comes to mind is a line from the script: "Fear blocks people's ears." Apparently, enormous relief does too.

❋

Performing in Kingston was magical for many reasons, but performing in Toronto was another thing again. For most of the cast, Toronto is where we live, where we work, where our connections and reputations really matter.

"And I thought I was scared in Kingston," Elaine says dryly.

Toronto is where Ross works.

He has always walked a fine line in his work, testing the limits of what will be tolerated in the bowels of biomedicine. Early in his career, he studied and wrote about patient advocacy, empowerment, and self-help groups—topics not always well received by medical colleagues.

But it was his leadership in writing a book about unconventional cancer therapies that got him in the most hot water. A friend called him a maverick. The new CEO called him irresponsible.

❋

It is 8 A.M. on November 25, 1998. The auditorium at Toronto Sunnybrook Regional Cancer Centre is dark. We can hear the shuffle and quiet conversation of nurses, physicians, administrative staff. Only the stage is lit. And we are on it, ready to begin.

And in walks the CEO.

"I was scared out of my gourd," says Mary Sue. "I thought, if we don't do it here, Ross is in trouble. I mean, we're up in front of the CEO, who's tough as nails, and these people who are going to crucify us if this doesn't come across. I didn't sleep that night."

Memorybank Drama: November 1998: Ross

Nothing in the research design courses I took at university prepared me for the moment that I stood in front of an audience at the hospital where I worked. My legs were shaking. I was convinced that I would fall to the floor. And I knew that all eyes in the auditorium were transfixed on my widely gyrating knees.

Sure, I had felt nervous presenting about research, but then I had notes to fall back on. I reflected wryly on the material, spoke dispassionately, stayed cool and distanced. Today, my task is to enter into an embodied form of research material and to portray it with passion. Vrenia has been after me to project more, to sell myself to the audience, to show them that I believe what I am saying in every pore of my body. It's not something I've ever done—or ever seen done—at Oncology Grand Rounds.

But that's not the whole of it. There's another kind of anxiety I experience with this event. It has to do with the tenuous nature of my professional survival, working in a health-care system that has shown little support over the years for social scientists—especially those who stray from mainstream approaches.

> I remember my first meeting with the CEO, who's sitting out there, towards the back. He told me I was behaving irresponsibly for leading a project that would better inform cancer patients about unconventional therapies. Another administrator—I can see him off to the left—handled the negotiations for the hospital several years ago, setting up my part-time contract after I and all the other members of the Psychology Department were laid off from full-time positions.
>
> Then there's the oncologist who fought on my behalf to ensure that the contract would be substantial enough for me to finish research projects I'd started before the layoff. And there's the head of research, a supporter of my gradual return to full-time status, a man who has stuck his neck out on my behalf. All of this feels very risky now.
>
> I look down again into the chasm of unemployment, the pain of rejection. What could possibly have possessed me to do this?

❋

The drama begins, and unfolds. There is not one moment in which it feels relaxed, not a second in which we have a sense of mastery of the script. If we could sell anxiety, this performance would make us all millionaires.

We reach the final scene. Ross and Patricia are seated, facing each other. Jan, Mary Sue, and Christina line up behind them, backs to the audience.

Ross, the doctor, looks at Patricia; there is nothing more he can do. "I'm sorry," he says, his words full with compassion. Patricia gasps, turns her head away.

Jan walks forward, circles around Patricia. Her voice is neutral, contained. "I am hormonal therapy, and I have nothing more to offer here." She walks between the two of them.

Christina follows suit. "I am radiation, and I have nothing more to offer here." Then Mary Sue: "I am chemotherapy, and I have nothing more to offer here." Christina circles again, more engaged: "I am your friend, and I am so distressed by what is happening to you, I have nothing more to offer here." She comes to a stop behind Patricia's chair.

Jan walks around Ross, her eyes focused on the "doctor": "I am seven years of training, residency, fellowship, books, research, articles, your white coat, your Medline searches—and I have nothing more to offer here." She stands behind his chair.

Mary Sue walks forward, stands between Patricia and Ross. "I am hope," she says, her arms extended in front of her. "Is there still room for me here?"

We can feel the hush in the audience.

Patricia's body shifts; she becomes an interviewer, curious, interested: "Doctor, how do you cope working with very ill patients?"

"I don't know," Ross responds. He turns, faces the audience. "Who says I'm coping?"

Memorybank Drama continued: November 1998: Ross

The auditorium is silent. And then the applause begins, tentative at first, then swelling to a roar. It goes on and on. We bow together. I can't stop smiling; am working at holding back tears. When the clapping finally ends, there is a moment of silence. A woman's voice emerges from the dark room. I recognize the head of Medical Oncology, one of the most prestigious breast cancer researchers in Canada.

"Don't turn up the lights," she says. "The doctors are crying." The auditorium erupts into laughter.

When the lights do come up, I see people dabbing at their eyes with tissues; others smiling broadly. Cast members introduce themselves, one by one. Then I cross the stage to

Jan with "information, information!" and Mary Sue as the doctor

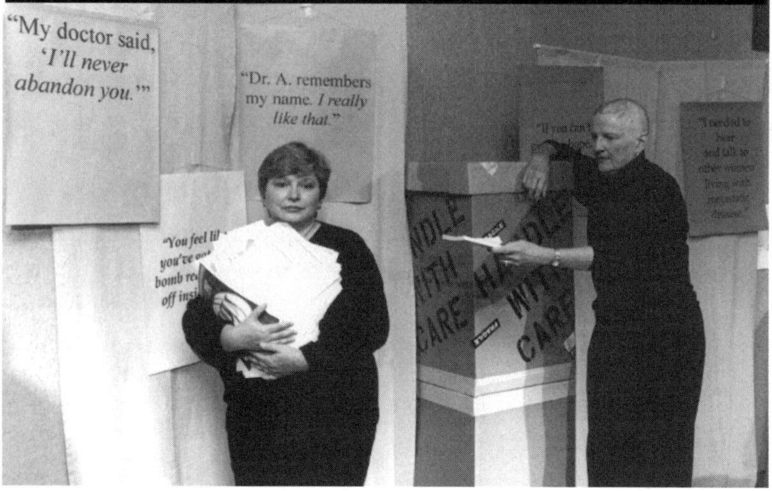
"My doctor said, 'I'll never abandon you.'"
"Dr. A. remembers my name. I really like that."

Vrenia leading our effort to come to grips with the research transcripts

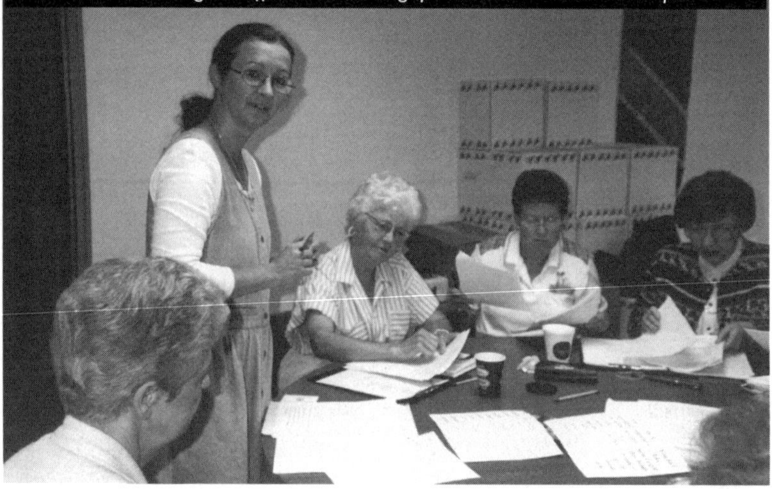

At a terribly tacky restaurant in Florida (yes, this photo is also a fridge magnet)

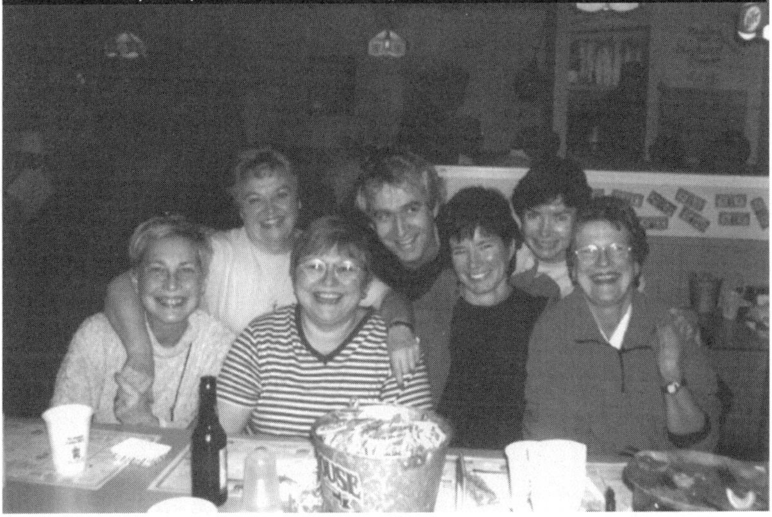

Hitting the big time in Jan's hometown

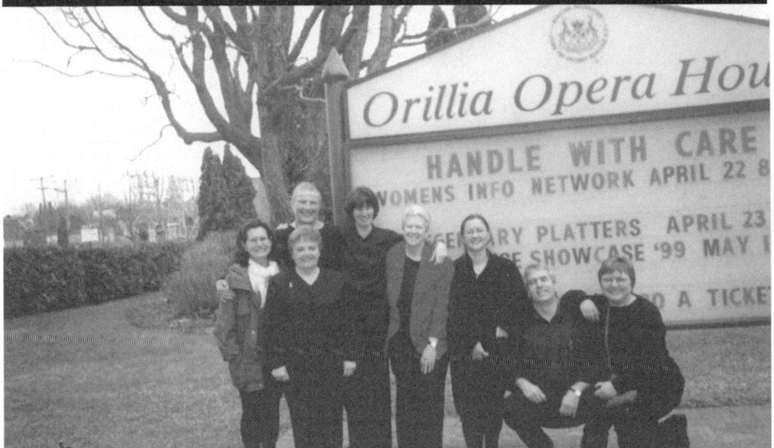

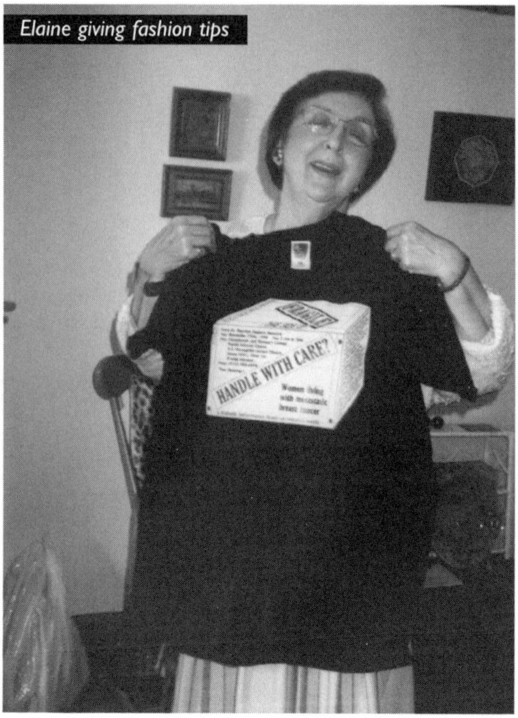

Elaine giving fashion tips

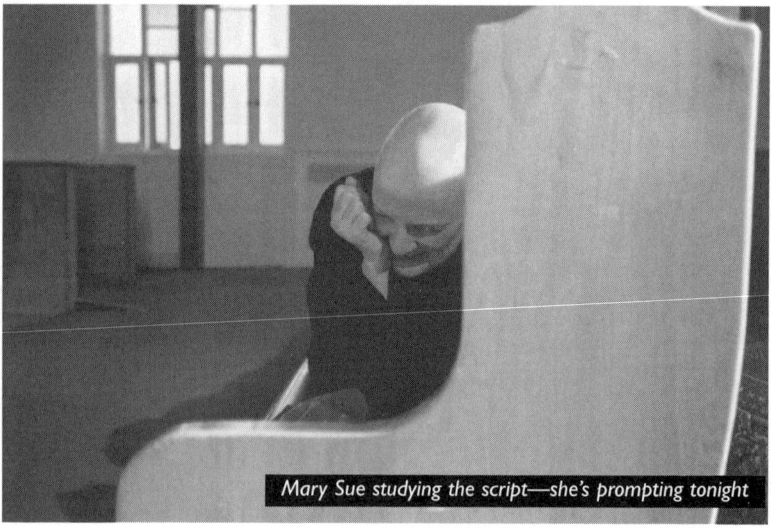

Mary Sue studying the script—she's prompting tonight

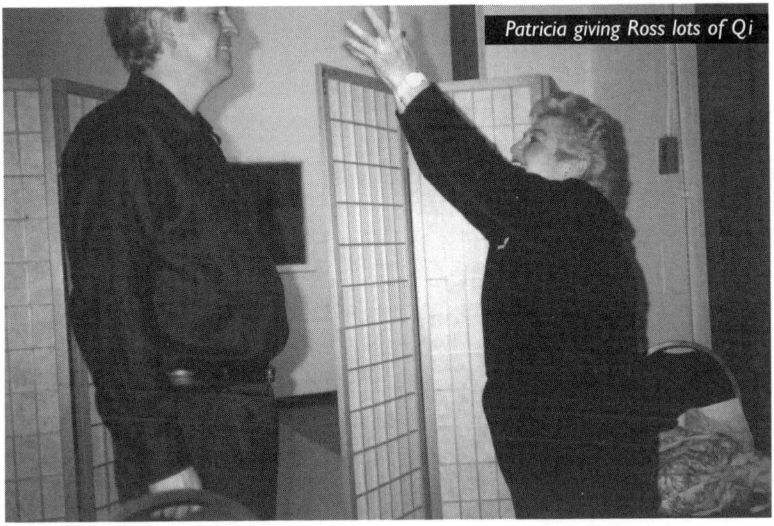

Patricia giving Ross lots of Qi

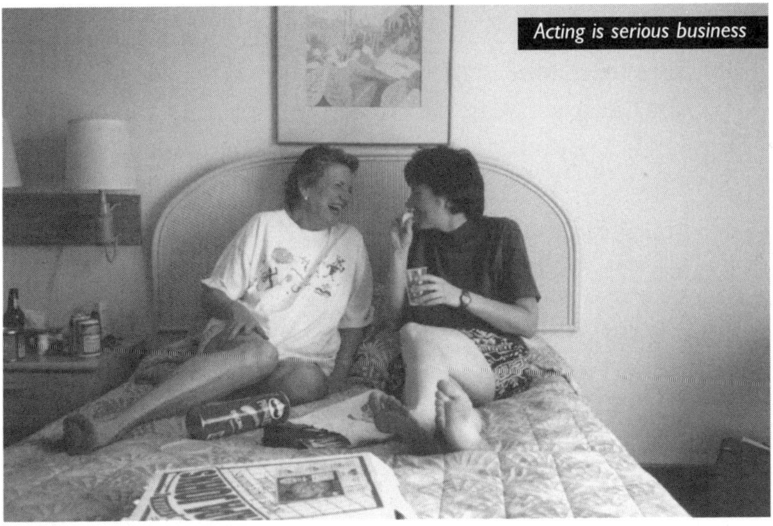

Acting is serious business

the lectern. In this moment, there is no memory of risk; all fear of failure is banished. How could I ever have doubted? I am limitless energy, boundless confidence. Later, Vrenia explains it to me. "That's what actors live for. Those moments."

Even in the thrall of postperformance headiness, I groan inside when I see the first hand that goes up. It's an oncologist who almost always asks the first question following Grand Rounds presentations. The question is inevitably intricate, inevitably difficult, usually focused on methodological limitations. The presenter—and it has been me on more than one occasion—is revealed for what s/he is: not nearly as bright as we all might have hoped.

I consider waiting for another hand, pretending not to see his, but then give in to the inevitability of it all. This is what I've been afraid of, this is the moment I've laid awake at night rehearsing. The questions about the validity of this type of presentation, the composition of the original research sample, the dissection of how—exactly how—we "translated" research to drama. I smile in his direction, welcome him to speak.

He stands. "I think this is a wonderful use of research. You are all to be commended . . . "

I don't hear what else he says. In this moment I know, absolutely know, that we are onto something important. Somehow, we've bypassed the analytic barriers, the habitual competitiveness. We've entered a new land. I am so thankful to be here.

There are other hands up. I call on people by name. An oncologist says that she was most struck by the family scenes. "You know, it's easy to forget how much cancer affects everyone in the family." Another oncologist laments about the struggles patients and doctors face in sorting through information about disease. "It's so hard for these patients. They get so much information and get so overwhelmed. And it just gets harder and harder for us to process it all with them. Do you have suggestions about what needs to happen?"

I explain that we have deliberately not been prescriptive in the play. "Our main concern is to reveal the difficulties surrounding issues of information. Clearly, there are no easy solutions, but we hope that the drama will motivate us all to keep struggling in finding the best ways to provide information for individual women."

A pharmacist asks about patients viewing the drama. "How do they react when they see the play?" I say that we've had a great response so far from women with breast cancer who've seen it. I recall comments we've heard from patients who say they better understand the dilemmas facing health professionals after seeing the drama. There is an appreciative hum in the audience. I say that patients are really curious about how health professionals respond to the play, that they like to hear that doctors are affected by it.

The CEO has his hand up. "This is a very important way of communicating information. Have you thought about taking it into medical schools?"

"We've thought about it, but haven't been able to arrange anything yet." I seize the chance to get a public commitment of support. "We'd welcome your help."

"I'd be glad to help." The next day, I ask him to write us a letter of commendation. He does, and it glows.

The discussion flows from one person to the next until I see the time is up. Afterwards, colleagues line up to talk about their reactions, extend their congratulations.

Comments also come back to us on evaluation forms we've distributed with the programs. "I've been giving chemotherapy for a number of years," wrote a nurse. "I've dealt with a lot of ladies with breast cancer. What struck me most about the play was, you see the other side of their lives, the kids, the husband not knowing exactly how to handle the situation, the frustration that goes along with illness. You forget about all of that, you're so focused on just making sure they know about the side effects of chemo."

A social worker wrote, "The messages came across loud and clear. As a health care provider, I was kind of bonked over the head, but in a very genuine way and in a way that didn't get my defenses up."

"The interplay of feelings of the patients and the medical professionals, rather than at war—that was really sensitively done," wrote another social worker. "They had different perspectives, obviously, but they weren't competitive or combative. And in some ways their feelings melded, they had the same feelings about some issues."

A month later, we performed in front of another health professional audience. An oncologist commented on a scene that emerged from one of the focus groups, about a woman's involvement in a clinical trial:

> B: I was part of the stem cell program, which is a wonderful program, and I tried so hard to do it for my doctor, to prove him, to be part of his statistics, and prove to other women that this is going to work and there's hope. And I didn't unfortunately do as well as we had hoped. And I felt like a failure. When I walked into the clinic, I didn't even want to look at the nurses, because I felt like such a failure. I've been spending all these months trying to deal with that.
>
> —From the *Handle with Care?* script

A physician in the audience said, "I'd never thought of that. A stem cell patient who does not respond and feels like a failure—that never occurred to me."

"I'm a resident here," said another man. "The whole premise of the research, 'handle with care'—that doesn't come across unless you actually see people dealing with it. Emotions don't come across in overheads or slides. Certainly they don't stay with you."

"I could see myself in this drama," another oncologist said. "I could see myself in the kind moments, and I could see myself in the asinine moments. We've all had lots of both."

❋

It is—still—November 25. Twelve hours later and we are at it again. Throngs of people are making their way into a huge auditorium, filling the seats. This is the hometown crowd, everyone's family members and friends.

We are waiting in the chapel. A few of us pace, shaking our arms as Jan has taught us. Ross widens his mouth into an "O," then puckers. This is a Vrenia exercise. We all join in, trying to limber our faces, ease the tension. It's not working.

"I am going to throw up," says Mary Sue.

She peers out of the room, watching the people entering the auditorium. Her husband, Peter, and three of their children are already seated. She sees another crowd of friends and clutches her stomach.

"I am really going to throw up," she says, and heads off—again—for the bathroom. She returns, and we walk together, shaking, into the room. Mary Sue manages to be gracious as she welcomes the crowd.

And then we begin. The audience is with us from the start, quick to laugh at all the right moments, rapt with attention.

Patricia moves to the front of the stage, starting the "Patient Guilt" scene. "Sometimes I think, is it because I've stayed in a bad marriage—is that why I have cancer?" she asks. "Not enough fresh vegetables? I should have had more. But I ate tons of broccoli!"

She turns slightly, looks into another part of the auditorium.

"Maybe it started when I was oil painting . . . the fumes." "The coffee," Jan interjects. "The chocolate," Christina says, accusingly. "The scotch," says Mary Sue—and a whole section of the auditorium bursts into laughter. Apparently, Mary Sue's fondness for scotch is neither exaggerated nor a secret.

We reach the "Hierarchy of Hope" and Mary Sue delivers her line. "I hope my husband learns to cook—better than he did last night." Laughter, and then a man's voice booms out from the audience. "Hey!" he says. "That's not in the script!" It is Peter, of course. Mary Sue laughs with him, and we finish the show.

After the performance, Mary Sue initiates a discussion with the audience. A woman several of us know from her volunteer work in the breast cancer community stands to speak.

"I was afraid to come tonight," she says. "I think it's true for a lot of us here—metastatic disease is our worst nightmare. But you did it with so much hope and so much humor. I really want to thank you for that."

A man in the audience agrees. "I think it has a stronger impact because it's a drama with comedy. If you had just been given the facts, they don't stay with you. They don't make such an impact."

"Were you there in his office, when I got the news?" one woman asks, referring to the diagnosis scene. "I mean, it was exactly like that!" Murmurs of recognition come from all corners of the room.

"My aunt's had cancer twice," says a twenty-something man near the front. "Everything that we've talked about was in the play. It was so accurate, so accurate! You feel like you'd know what to say, what to do, if anything came up in your own family."

A young woman puts her hand up. "My mother has breast cancer," she says. "Everything that went on in the play was what we are going through, even down to how the brother was reacting. I wasn't around a lot when my mom was first diagnosed. . . ." Tears slide into her voice. "I feel like I know more now, what it was like for her." She sits down and the woman beside her puts an arm over her shoulder, kisses her cheek.

"There was a kind of realness about the things I was hearing," someone says from the front row. "I know that was because several of you have experienced cancer. I know the lines were rehearsed, but it didn't feel like a rehearsed drama as much as some people coming together taking about their experiences. I think patients can relate to this better than to a big fancy drama."

Researcher Rant: August 2000: Ross

From the outset of this project, my central concern was that *Handle with Care?* reflect issues that women with metastatic breast cancer, and the people around them, would recognize from their experiences. Accomplishing this would mean that we had effectively carried the findings of our original research forward into the drama. The feedback we got from audiences provided the consensual validity I was seeking. But I had another hope, ultimately more important—that the drama would affect people who saw it in ways that helped them.

None of the numerous applied and participatory projects I have been involved with over the past dozen years have come close to having the impact of *Handle with Care?* The postmodern act of revealing the different perspectives of ill women, health professionals, and family members turned out to be immensely meaningful, even "transformative," for audience members. People are hungry for authentic representations of important aspects of their lives, such as living with illness. The insights reported by audience members at *Handle with Care?* performances reverberate in daily life.

At first, I was resistant to the thought of launching a more in-depth investigation of the impact of research-based drama. I mean, I didn't need any more convincing of positive value beyond the immediate responses of our audiences. But I work in an environment steeped in the rituals of systematic, evidence-based evaluation. Eventually, I turned towards the possibility of assessing its impact, but, because of the timing of things, we decided to undertake an evaluative study after *Handle with Care?* ended, as part of our next drama project, *No Big Deal?*

The notion of studying impact is complicated. The physician who suggested we target specific physician attitudes and behaviors and look for postperformance shifts didn't really understand what we had done. Our focus was on portraying the lived experiences of women (and others), not on affecting behaviors. How could we then expect to track specific behavioral change?

In preparing to write a proposal for the evaluation study, I did a series of interviews with people I work with, to try and understand how *Handle with Care?* had affected them. All of them described an ongoing impact of the performance, but none spoke about that impact primarily in terms of behavioral change or new learning. Several physicians described the importance of being reminded of the struggles of ill people, and of the network of people connected to them. One physician described, in detail, scenes of the performance that she often recalls during busy clinics, scenes that help to remind her of the impact her words have on patients. Another physician said that she was able to see more deeply into issues that she had already understood intellectually. Although she was unsure if this had implications for her behavior, she wondered if she was more caring in how she goes about her usual tasks. A nurse stated that the importance of the performance for her was the "revealing" of the health professionals' world to patients and vice versa. She felt that seeing the performance helped counteract the ever-present possibility of burnout for health professionals like her. She also described how a breast cancer patient, after seeing the performance, had reported to her how ecstatic she was that her family and friends were given a window through which to see the challenges she was facing in her life. Another nurse said it was critically important to break through the barriers that health professionals construct to protect themselves, but which make them emotionally unavailable to their patients.

Whereas these informants didn't think about the impact of drama in terms of their own behavioral change or learning, several commented that this might be different for other groups, such as spouses, other family members, or friends of ill people. They suggested that any investigation of impact cover a wide range of possibilities, including, but not limited to, behavioral change.

So I wrote the proposal as a qualitative study, aiming to explore in depth the many facets of audience member responses to a research-based drama. I wasn't sure how the proposal would be received, given the strong biases within social science intervention research—that only specific behavioral changes are legitimate evidence of a useful intervention, and then only as proven through randomized clinical trials. But the proposal was approved, and funded by the National Cancer Institute of Canada.

But let me move away from the formal approach to evaluating the merit of our drama work. During the last interview Christina conducted with me, we were speculating, once again, on what it all meant; you know, the big picture.

Earlier in our conversation, Christina had been talking about a preschool in Zimbabwe that she was involved in supporting—in the midst of political and social chaos, in the midst of an AIDS epidemic, this one initiative to try and help children get a leg up. Would it, could it, really make a difference? Was it yet another well-intentioned, but ultimately empty, attempt to alleviate unnecessary suffering?

"You know what you were saying about Zimbabwe, and that question about what's really worth doing," I said in the interview. "And how from one perspective, you can look at this effort, this attempt to make things better, and it seems to just disappear, swallowed up by all the other forces that swirl around. You know, the zeitgeist is just too powerful, too negative. And I think it's that way with *Handle with Care?* too. The health care system, the whole North American society, is so twisted away from compassion. Did we really think we could change all of that? But, it's like something still happens. In the middle of all this health system reorganization, cutting back of services, clinical trials, health professional burnout, there is this drama—it becomes visible, travels, evokes people's feelings about all the pain they live with, all the hopes they once had to make a difference. It shines a light on everything that's going on. It's really quite astonishing."

❃

CHAPTER SEVEN
WE BEHAVED BADLY

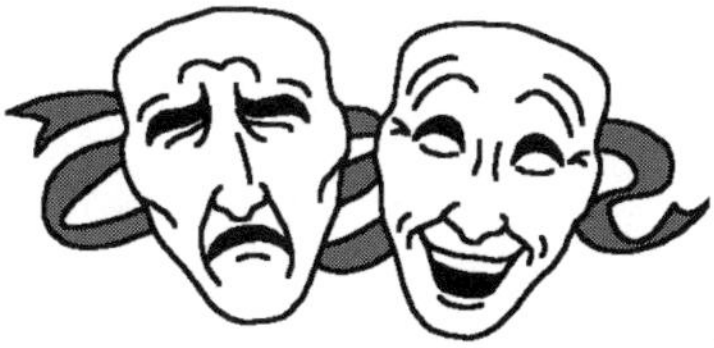

As we were developing the *Handle with Care?* script, we spent several sessions focusing on physician perspectives. We were looking for ways to represent the demands of an oncologist's daily work, to capture some of the challenges they face in interactions with patients.

Vrenia taught us to create "statues," to silently organize our bodies to express a particular moment or meaning. In one, Ann was the doctor, trying to swim through a maze of barriers and obstacles. In another, Mary Sue had her head down on a desk, protecting herself from various people tugging and prodding at her. We each walked around the statues, commenting on them, assessing what they conveyed about an oncologist's realities. Then Vrenia switched gears; we moved into improvisation.

In one improv, Jan played the role of a doctor valiantly attempting to concentrate on a colleague's article. Her nurse interrupted constantly: the doctor's son had called to remind her about his hockey game, a patient's blood-work results needed follow up, the doctor's mother had been taken to a hospital. Another physician appeared, insisting that a research paper required immediate completion. Into this welter of demands rolled Mrs. Yammer.

"My Son's Mother-in-Law's Brother Is a Doctor" from the *Handle with Care?* Script

(MRS. YAMMER (C) ENTERS WITH BAGS OF BOOKS, ARTICLES, AND PAPER)

B DOC: Come on in, Mrs. Yammer. I'll be with you in just a moment.

(MRS. YAMMER SITS. STARTS SORTING THROUGH BAGS)

B DOC: All right then. How have you been since our last appointment?

C MRS. Y: Not too well actually. But on my good days I've been doing all sorts of research. I picked up a book at the health food store [SEARCHES FOR IT]. Now where is it? Well, it talks about shark cartilage for cancer. Have you heard of it? Sharks don't get cancer, you know. The health food store says they can't keep up with the demand. It might be worth trying. And then this neighbor of mine says her sister who's got stomach cancer was told she had six weeks to live and a year later her cancer's gone because she went to Quebec to do a juice fast. I even found something on the Internet about it. [SEARCHES AND PULLS OUT LONG SHEETS].

A NURSE: [ENTERING] Excuse me, Doctor. Here's the fax you wanted. These forms need your signature right away. [DOCTOR SIGNS. NURSE LEAVES]

C MRS. Y: And this may be just the thing. There was an article in the paper about this new drug. There are clinical trials somewhere—Oh, where is it? Well, I'm sure you read it. You know, Doctor, my son's mother-in-law's brother is a doctor and he's a bit distressed with the course of treatment you've got me on. He doesn't think you're tackling this aggressively enough.

B DOC: And what is his field?

C MRS. Y: He's a veterinarian. But they do know a lot about nutrition. And animals get cancer too, you know!

(DOCTOR PUTS HEAD ON DESK)

As Vrenia remembers it, the "Mrs. Yammer" improvisation marked "the first time we got into really raucous laughter, where we were rolling on the floor. We discovered a truth about the doctor's world that inspired our compassion. And I think it released us from the holiness of the subject of cancer, too. Mrs. Yammer was a cancer patient, and we could laugh at her, at the same time feeling compassion for the thing that was driving her to behave the way she was. I don't think after that anything was sacred."

The reverential quality of our engagement with cancer—and our shift to another kind of response to metastatic disease and the people with it—was something Elaine also noticed.

"When you are dealing with someone with an illness," she said, "you are very careful of your jokes. When we are talking about death as much as life, you're, I think, subconsciously guarded, unless somehow or other you've been able to establish the feeling that anything goes, in the kindest sense."

In the end, as well, it was our laughter that confirmed to Jan that we had acquired the knowledge about metastatic disease that, for her, counted as knowledge. "When we all belly-laughed for the first time, and I don't even know what caused it, but the real sense of hilarity—and everybody was laughing and I thought: 'They've got it, they've got it! You can have this fucking disease—and you can still laugh.'"

As the drama moved across the province in the fall of 1998, people who had seen or heard about the show called Ross to explore the possibility of additional performances. As the new year approached, the few requests had become a steady stream.

Ross and Vrenia conferred. Our plan had been to wrap up in April 1999. But perhaps we could go into the fall? A few things were certain: If we did extend performances, we would need a larger pool of actors to draw from. And Ross and Christina could not possibly continue to do all the organizing. We would need to hire someone. We would need more money.

Researcher Rant: August 2000: Ross

Hustling is not new to those of us engaged with grantsmanship. But research-based theater demands hustling on an entirely new level.

Funding for the original studies on which *Handle with Care?* and *No Big Deal?* were based came from major research funding agencies. But we thought it unlikely that these same agencies would approve funding to mount and travel a theater production as part of a research grant. To be honest, fearing rejection and the interminable wait for said rejection, we did not pursue this path. Instead, we turned directly to cancer organizations and corporations.

In the beginning, we were fortunate enough to receive an education grant from the Canadian Breast Cancer Foundation, which provided for some of the initial costs of mounting the *Handle with Care?* production. But we had to proceed on faith, hoping other funds would be forthcoming. Eventually, after we had been performing for several months, and fearing we would not have the money to meet our accumulating commitments, more funding was provided.

We would not have been able to get the production on its feet without additional support from corporate sponsors. Wheeling and dealing in this unfamiliar terrain made for a steep learning curve. I quickly realized that sponsorship (from corporations and cancer organizations alike) is only partially related to the quality of a "product." It is also related to what can be provided to sponsors—acknowledgement, profile, access to potential purchasers and clients. I gathered logos and sent company representatives *Handle with Care?* t-shirts.

It was a whole new set of criteria by which to be judged. Nobody in the corporate world cared about the rigor of our methodology, or whether there was a strong theoretical basis for the work. They cared about selling things. They cared about influencing physicians' prescribing patterns. They cared about image. More and more, I came to care about these things too.

It is not that I want to be caring about them. I do not believe that consumerism should be the guiding principal of our society. But I don't run this world.

Part of me cringes at the new entrepreneurial heights (depths?) that these projects have demanded of me. Some days, I remind myself of the aluminum siding salesmen in Tin Men, a Richard Dreyfuss and Danny DeVito comedy. At what point does the admired entrepreneurial hustler become a con man? Where are the ethical guidelines to chart my path? More than one pharmaceutical representative wondered aloud if I might be persuaded to insert the name of their drug into the dialogue of a show. I've said no. So far.

I did my best to woo wealthy patrons, not much liking the role—even when I was successful. I winced when a colleague reported that an eventual donor to the project confided to her that I was "a good beggar."

I admit that there is also part of me that gets charged up about my newfound need to seek financial support outside the sheltered halls of academe and government-sponsored granting agencies. Too much reliance on traditional research funding sources can lead researchers to believe that approval of peers through review processes is proof of relevance and social value. And accountability too easily gets framed in terms of final budget reports and appropriate profiling of granting agencies in peer-reviewed publications.

I was terrified to try and compete in the open market, but I also found it refreshing to be so accountable. We are accountable to our sponsors, but that is secondary to our accountability to audiences. If we are not providing a product that gets them excited, that makes a difference in their lives, we will not be in business for long.

❃

When Ross and Vrenia came to the decision to extend the *Handle with Care?* schedule, Ross sought out an administrator and Vrenia went in search of more actors. Fran Turner came aboard as "coordinator, research-based theater" (a title perhaps unique in the universe at this juncture in time), and Vrenia approached several members of Act II Studio to see if they would be involved. In the late fall of 1998, rehearsals began—again.

Having to work up a new cast was difficult at first, Vrenia explained to Ross one day. Partly it was the repetition, walking through the scenes over and over again, after having gone through them—over and over again—with the first troupe. But it was hard for other reasons.

"It's a funny thing," Vrenia said. "I felt isolated. And I had resentment—because, I thought, these people have no relationship whatsoever to any of us here, and they haven't been through what we've been through. And having not gone through the experience, of course, they treated the script as if it were religious material. They were so maudlin with it all, and it felt awful. I also felt very protective of our material because it wasn't just my material, it wasn't just a play. Our hearts and souls had gone into creating the script. And I guess I was also really proud."

Ross and Vrenia decided to organize a meeting where new cast members could see the original troupe perform *Handle with Care?* Vrenia remembers the day it happened.

"I was really looking forward to the original cast coming in and showing the new cast how to do it—and showing them, I think, the energy. I wanted them to really feel the defiance in the energy of the group. And what happened instead"—Vrenia pauses, laughs—"is that we were all so delighted to see each other that we were like a bunch of two-year-olds reintroduced at the day care."

Elaine picks up the story. "As people walked into the room, there was this great, joyous hugging. And these poor guys—the new cast—sat in a row, stunned, behind the table."

"We got up there to do the show," Patricia remembers, "and everyone thinks this wonderful cast is coming on—and I couldn't remember the first line!"

"The group was very undisciplined," says Vrenia. "And I guess it had been a while since people had done the show—and they were terrible. And they were all laughing. I kept thinking, 'Oh, what a horrible director I am to allow this amount of undisciplined activity!'"

"We really did behave badly," says Mary Sue.

"I think it was borderline rude, if you want to know the truth," says Elaine, with her famous raised brow.

Of course, we all have our own theories about why that meeting went as it did. "I think what it is—we miss each other, when we're away from each other." Vrenia leans forward, explaining it. "I think what I really missed was the laughter, because laughter, a certain quality of laughter, a very raucous laughter, had always been part of our experience. So, when the original group came in, we all wanted to hug, we were all missing the laughter, we were missing what we had."

"We were so glad to be together, so that was part of it," Mary Sue remembers. "We'd always laughed a lot and it was wonderful to have those great laughs. You don't have those too often, just flat-out hysterical laughter."

She pauses, thinks about it some more. "I think it was partly, too, saying: 'This is serious, but there is some fun here too.' I think we looked at them, the new actors, and it seemed so traumatic, sad and awful. Part of that release for us was to show them that this is not what it is. We'd been through that, the statistics and stuff, and then we did learn to move on, and laugh, and go on from there."

"In the beginning, it seemed to be such a—oh, a dire subject, a doom-and-gloom subject, that we had to at some point bring some laughter into it," Patricia explains. "And we'd grown on that. We were comfortable enough that we could joke about things without taking anything away from the whole project. I think the new cast was a little surprised that we were making such a joyful thing of it. But it was important for them to see that because, yes, it is a doom-and-gloom subject, but you have to realize that there has to be some laughter and some hope with it too."

"I think one way of dealing with the work," says Vrenia, "is to constantly make jokes, and notice the ironies in the language, and be playful with it. We have a tendency to build on top of one another that way."

"I think it was territorial," Elaine declares. "Like wolves and dogs mark their area. Some of us knew we were going a bit overboard in nonsense. There was almost, on the old cast's part, a 'Yeah, we've suffered. We've created this, we've suffered, we've done it all, you know—and look at us, we're having sort of a good time.' And it could jolly well have been, if we're really honest, a good bit of nervousness on our part! It's okay with audiences, but when you perform for somebody who is going to take your place, then you're on an equal basis. I think the other group has been very kind in liking us and tolerating us," she concludes firmly.

Over time, of course, the new cast mixed in with the original group, joining in with the laughter. Our laughter marked our connections to one another, but it was laughter very much in the midst of and in relation to the more difficult passages we had traveled over the course of creating *Handle with Care?*

Early on in our work as a group, Mary Sue found our persistent attention to her illness quite unsettling. "I've found it much more difficult than I thought I would, in that I can separate out this metastatic disease from my life most of the time. And coming here and having to deal with it, and bring it up in my mind, and vocally, for two hours or three hours, has brought it to the surface. It has been difficult for me because I've come home and thought about it a lot, and had trouble sleeping sometimes at night after I'd been there."

For the women who were part of Act II Studio who have had breast cancer, participating in *Handle with Care?* foregrounded the possibility of their own disease recurring. "I had breast cancer; it was a horror," one woman said. "As quickly as I could, I put it away. I have absolutely no desire to meet and talk about breast cancer with anybody, and I certainly have no desire to hear, over and over again, 'I was clear for ten years and then it returned.' Every time I hear something of that kind, it's like a stab which I do not need and do not want."

"Being involved with Mary Sue and Jan, and having had breast cancer myself," Patricia said, "things start to worry you a little bit more, you know, that you're never free of it. I mean, I always assumed I was free of it—hopefully I am, that is the way I look at it, I don't dwell on it. But you know there's always that little grain of fear there."

For Patricia, participating in the development of *Handle with Care?* heightened her vigilance around possible signs of metastasis and intensified an uneasy internal dialogue.

"I still have a three-month supply of [a drug intended to prevent recurrence] in my drawer, and I go look at it now and again and think—especially since I've been involved with this group—should I take those pills again? I sort of covered the bottle up but then, you know, I've gone back and looked at it. Maybe it's kind of like a blanket. I think, 'Oh maybe I should wrap that blanket around me again,' and then I think, 'What's the point? What good is three months going to do me?' But it's there anyway."

Another actor who had experienced a breast cancer diagnosis described women like Patricia and herself as the ones "in the middle," trapped, in one sense, between the people in the group who had not had cancer, and the women who had metastatic disease. "The ones in the middle," she said "you've got the next step—metastatic disease—which might not come, it's not inevitable, but if it comes, that's it, there's no defense. Especially, don't forget that it's we who have already fought a battle and presumably won, because we are still there. And having won it, and feeling we can go on with our lives, and suddenly we're faced with 'Oh, you think you've won, but not necessarily.'"

For some women with a primary diagnosis, engaging in this project was a kind of ongoing admonishment about the impossibility of security in their futures. At the same time, as Patricia said, "If it did happen to me [a recurrence], I think, probably because of this experience, I would handle it much better. I think I'd have to—because of Mary Sue and Jan. I'd want to be involved differently, know more, do more."

Particular moments in the drama's development, like the statistics meeting, were hard for everyone in the troupe, for different reasons. Ann also talked about how difficult it was for some people to read the transcripts of interviews with physicians.

"I think both Jan and Mary Sue, in reading the oncologist transcripts, probably felt quite vulnerable," she said. "It's not spoken as if there is a patient listening. And particularly the oncologist who was so compassionate, I mean, I felt vulnerable reading that. I didn't expect that; the breath is caught. For the patient to enter that sensibility was to feel quite vulnerable. When we're scared, we really want the people we're depending on to be safe. We want to know that they won't be harmed by this too."

Researcher Rant: August 2000: Ross

I think that one expression of research ethics is researcher worry. I worried about the actors in *Handle with Care?* Several of the women who were initially treated for breast cancer feared a recurrence as we read transcripts about the experience of metastatic disease. What right had we, as researchers, to introduce this into their lives? Another woman talked about her nightmares about a possible first diagnosis. Would she be okay? And then I worried about Jan and Mary Sue. How long could they stay well? Did they feel that their incredible efforts on behalf of this project were worthwhile? How would the other actors be affected if one of them suddenly became critically ill, or died? How does informed consent apply to potential actors, in this kind of context? How is consent best enacted?

In both *Handle with Care?* and *No Big Deal?* I worried about our audiences. Were there some women who had been told they had metastatic cancer, but never been told it is incurable? Would we inadvertently undermine hope and send individual women careening into crisis? Watching *No Big Deal?* would some men be shamed by our joking about sex, or feel a new sense of inadequacy when they saw how others have been willing to communicate, willing to reach out to the women in their lives?

Thinking carefully about the cast and audience members, trying to anticipate, and worrying about, their responses to the drama—these are gestures in the direction of ethical practice. And always these gestures can be made extravagant. Taking care with others' feelings and experiences can shade into a fantasy about our own power, and a construction of all who take part in the drama as victims, unable to resist its impact. It is also an ethical stance to assert that people can and will take care of themselves.

In both dramas, we wrestled—with ourselves and with one another—to find an ethical place where we could stand, more or less together. The publicity material we created for *Handle with Care?* clearly stated that the drama spoke to the experiences of women with *metastatic* breast cancer. In most instances, we defined metastatic. We wanted everyone to know what he or she was getting into. Later, people who had seen the performance became its ambassadors, and the responsibility we felt for representing the drama in a way that attended to its potentially difficult effects diminished.

In the introduction to the drama, we note that "while metastatic disease is rarely curable, it can be treated, and many people in communities around Ontario are living with it today." The phrase emphasizes that medicine can and does respond to the illness, and affirms a community of people living with it. This seemed important when we wrote the introduction, and still does. Other choices we might now (but didn't at the time) consider in the realm of ethics are embedded in the staging. One woman who saw the drama remarked on the ways the choreography of the drama moved people towards hard places, then carried them away as the next scene transformed the tone and the players. "You got sad," she said, "but you didn't stay there."

As we began working on *No Big Deal?* we also talked more formally with potential actors about the risks and benefits of their participation. Yet new issues arose, and we continue to grapple with many thorny ethical issues on the fly. Like others working in this fledgling field, I feel an urgency to sort them through to avoid unnecessary mistakes, unnecessary suffering.

Researcher Rant: August 2000: Christina

In my mind, the experiences of the women with a primary breast cancer diagnosis raised most urgently the ethical questions in *Handle with Care?* Women with breast cancer were profoundly implicated in all of our discussions and investigations about metastatic disease. They were always, in very difficult ways, "understudies" for Mary Sue and Jan's "roles." Yet, as is the case with understudies, their experiences were never the primary focus of our attention.

If the process of creating *Handle with Care?* had been conceptualized as a research undertaking, questions around its impact on participants would likely have been framed in terms of harm and risk (Miles and Huberman 1994). Some of the risks taken in the course of the project were quite publicly acknowledged. Others were more privately explored. In relation to the women with a primary diagnosis, Ann speculated that they might "go away with more vulnerability about their illness than they had. I think that's probably inevitable."

In this setting, perhaps more clearly than in most qualitative research undertakings, women with a primary diagnosis were expected not only to speak about but also to witness, to enter into, to take on, their possible future. As actors, they were required to study for, and enact, a part. As "understudies" in a much more profound sense, they were asked to understand the role "woman with metastatic disease" and to anticipate the possibility that they may someday be required to live it. In future projects, we will no doubt attend more carefully to the precarious position of the understudy.

At the same time, many research approaches—participatory models, for instance—challenge traditional ethical frameworks. In discussing anonymity, the assurance of which is generally assumed to be standard ethical practice, Miles and Huberman (1994) note that in action or collaborative research, participants may well want to be credited for their work. In a parallel way, participatory and collaborative approaches may prompt us to rethink assumptions about "harm."

One woman with a primary diagnosis confirmed that participating in *Handle with Care?* was, at times, immensely difficult for her. She also noted that the particular struggles women in her situation faced in the project were relatively unremarked. But, she also pointed out that "the fact that one isn't supported, and the fact that this is unpleasant, doesn't necessarily mean that one has to leave. . . . I'm glad that I hung in there."

Jan, reflecting on the project, spoke about being "bothered" at times by the focus on metastatic disease. As she went on to say, however, "sometimes when I'm peeling the potatoes I get bothered too. I'm never really away from thoughts that sort of just crop up and make me sad, or make me wonder what my future is.

"In some ways," Jan continued, "my involvement in this drama helped crystallize some of those thoughts. Like the one scene I suggested to Vrenia around the diagnosis, that was so clear to me. It wasn't clear to me before I started this. I hadn't thought about it in terms of how I could present that to other people. I knew how I felt in that moment and that was all that was important and now, okay, how do I make other people understand how I felt? It really just helped to crystallize it. In some ways, that's been good. I can put my finger on my ideas a little faster or explain them to other people."

Being involved in *Handle with Care?* was, for Jan, "an opportunity to say things out loud and try them on. 'How's that feel?' or 'Gee, I made that sound worse than it really is, how can we fix this?'" She described gaining a different perspective on her illness, and a certain kind of ease.

"I am thinking about my diagnosis more, but I am also more comfortable in my shoes in that I have been given an opportunity to explore some of what I am afraid of. To tell other people what I am afraid of, to tell them things they could do differently that would be helpful to me or whatever. This play has sort of allowed me to visit those sad feelings, those angry feelings, the feelings of disappointment, being ripped off—all sorts of things."

She paused, reflecting on it. "It has made me less afraid," she said finally. "The bottom line is, I don't want to die, not yet, and not soon. I have a lot of things I want to do. I want to know my daughter is loved and comfortable in her adult life and, you know, all those sorts of things. And when will she be comfortable in her adult life? Maybe when she's fifty? Or I'm seventy-six? And I don't like to think about dying on a regular basis, but in this, doing this show somehow, articulating, and saying these words out loud—maybe I'm an auditory learner, I don't know . . . but saying things out loud, and sort of manipulating them with my mind and my mouth . . . you know?"

Here, Jan spoke again about the diagnosis scene. In the drama, Jan often plays the patient devastated by the results of her bone scan. Three other characters stand behind her to represent the voices in her head. The voices insist that she not faint, that she "breathe!"

"I really listen in the diagnosis scene because it helps get me where I need to go. I'm really concentrating. You know when you say 'breathe' the first time, I feel my lungs swell up. I listen. I don't know. Somehow it's okay, it's . . . comforting for a minute."

In the context of her engagement with the rest of the troupe, and her "performing" of metastatic disease, Jan's illness was transformed into something she took hold of, something she grasped differently than she had before. As she focused on how to dramatize critical moments and emotions, her experience of metastatic disease became more tangible—her feelings crystallized, she could more quickly put her finger on ideas—and its essence was more clearly apprehended; it became something she could stage, choreograph, present.

Even further, in saying out loud words like "dying" as she rehearsed and performed, she had a sense of manipulating her most profoundly threatening thoughts. Metastatic disease became sayable-out-loud, became less "unspeakable," less inexpressibly awful. In a certain way, it became "presentable." As Park-Fuller (2000, 24) suggests, "in acts of telling, speakers often come to understand events in new ways—in ways of their own construction." In a similar vein, Mary Sue noted that "performing in front of so many people without my hair, has made it much easier to be without my hair." Exposed repeatedly and to hundreds of people in performance, her bare head became less uneasily bare in her daily life.

Of course, the thoughts that make Jan sad or make her wonder about her future still "crop up." The meaning of metastatic disease as anguish, as profound and unpredictable disruption, was not erased by *Handle with Care?* The comfort she identified was, after all, "for a minute." Yet through the scene she was central to creating, she articulated those thoughts, and she had us embody them, make them "solid"; and, in performance, she anticipates and listens intently to them for her own reasons rather than having them manifest without warning and against her will. The thoughts that often define a woman's experience of living with the disease can, in this context and for this moment, be changed—by artful means—to serve her own purposes.

Memorybank Drama: October 1998: Christina

We are loading two cars outside of some hospital—is it Chatham? We are, I think, pleased with ourselves, with how the performance has gone. The two cars will travel different routes: Ross will take Patricia and Mary Sue back to Toronto, I will drop Jan off on my way home to Dundas.

Jan and I hug Patricia and Mary Sue goodbye. Affection glows amongst this circle of women. Jan looks over at Ross. "You know what? I am going to hug that man."

Decisive, she makes her way over, folds him in her arms. From this moment on, Ross is huggable.

Researcher Rant: August 2000: Ross

I value collegiality and have enjoyed my involvement with (most) other researchers over the years. But no previous research project plunged me so far into the intimacies of social relationships as *Handle with Care?* My usual task-focused way limits the amount of airtime given to personal material. Research is, after all, about getting things done. But that would not do with these women. They wanted to know about me. And not just the kind of studies I do.

At first, I resisted. But as time went on, I moved to meet my new companions more on their own terms. Their terms have more to do with friendship than collaboration. More to do with sharing than information. More to do with intimacy and vulnerability than boundaries. By their behavior, this group rejected all conventions of distance that are constructed for and by researchers. They insisted on reciprocity, and they challenged and sometimes even manipulated me to embrace their assumptions. I now believe this approach was integral to our project's success.

The day following our stunningly successful Toronto debut of *Handle with Care?* several members of the group called me. They all said how happy they were for me, to have taken such an enormous risk with the project and that it paid off. I was taken aback, not expecting such warmth, such personal attention. I am grateful.

❃

"Do you know what's amazing to me?" Mary Sue asked Christina one day. "The other women from Act II Studio, and how much they have taken *Handle with Care?* into their hearts and been part of it. I can see it for me, I can see it for Jan, and for you and Ross, but these people came from out there. And have really bought in and loved it as much as we have."

Phyllis, a longtime member of Act II Studio, remembers what it was like when she first met Mary Sue and Jan.

"The part about treating them differently—it's like the Magda scene. Until you know they have this disease, they're sort of the same as you. And then, when you know, you put on kid gloves and you sort of look at them through a cloud. And that's the way a lot of us, including myself, have been doing it, worrying: 'What do I say?' This project has changed my approach. It's given me insight that I wouldn't have had."

Sandra said that being involved in the drama "helped me deal with people who have serious illness and understand the effect on everyone. I want to try and treat people 'real-ly', to be sensitive to how they see and hear things."

"One still often travels in the dark in trying to be supportive to a friend," Elaine said. "You just don't know what the best thing is. But I think that I've had increased courage to venture more."

Working on *Handle with Care?* also generated an extraordinary sense of achievement for people. "I have loved being part of seeing something develop and creating something," said Mary Sue. Jan agreed. "It is exciting to be part of something that is new. It is also trying and emotionally, physically, mentally exhausting, but I think the goal is worth it," she said.

The sense of achievement has a particular meaning for Jan in the context of her prognosis. "Every time we get to the 'Hierarchy of Hope' scene and say, 'I hope people don't forget me'—that was the line I gave and I think there's a part of that. If my time is limited and it probably is . . . is this my last chance to make a mark on the world? I don't think so, but, you know . . . "

CHAPTER EIGHT
BLOCKING NOTES

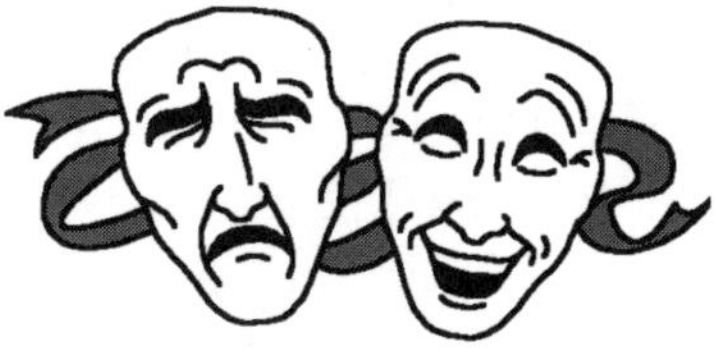

We are, once again, at the Sunnybrook Cancer Centre. Milling about in the hallway outside of the room where we had our first Toronto audience with health professionals, we catch up with one another's lives, tell stories about the first season of performances, fill up on coffee and muffins. It is June 1999.

The purposes of our gathering are many and various. Fran, who is orchestrating the hive of research-based theater activity now buzzing at Sunnybrook, wants to map out the next year of performances and distribute schedules. We need to discuss the introduction of new actors and review the funding situation. Then everyone will have lunch, and the people who have been part of the project from the beginning will stay for the afternoon. We've planned an opportunity to reflect about the past months and discuss the themes that have emerged from interviews with this group. Ross and Christina want to see if the directions they're taking in writing about *Handle with Care?* ring true with the people who took part in those interviews and who made the drama possible.

Ross takes us through the morning session and at noon Christina is sitting on the floor munching away on grilled vegetables when Jan kneels carefully beside her. "Have you heard about Mary Sue?" "No," Christina says. "What?"

"The tumors in her lungs have grown," Jan says grimly. "She's starting treatment again."

Christina groans. The anguish is back.

Jan and Christina talk for a while, and then have to hurry towards the next session. The troupe filters into the room, still chattering and eating. Christina stands, turns to face them.

"Okay," she says. "This is the moment when all those conversations I had with you, with my tape recorder between us, come together." She tells everybody that she has selected quotes from the interviews and those quotes now line the hallway outside the room. "Because I'm moving house," she says, "the quotes are taped to packing paper." She explains that the quotes are organized to describe what it took for the group to create *Handle with Care?*

"I want you to think about the flow of ideas here," Christina instructs. "See if the movement of them seems true to you, because they are going to guide how we write about this project. If you look at the quotes and think, 'Were you in the same room we were, Christina? Perhaps you were working on the prostate project?'—that's a problem, that's something we need to know. If there's anything missing, if any important component of what it took for us as a group to create this drama isn't captured there, we need to know that too."

"Once we've had a chance to look at the quotes," she continues, "we'll come back and talk about them. And I want to spend some time exploring what we learned about research-based theater—what we would have done differently, what we would tell other people who might embark on a research-based theater journey. How does all that sound?"

"I think it's perfect they're on packing paper," Mary Sue smiles, "for *Handle with Care?*"

Everyone laughs. "I hadn't thought about that," Christina exclaims. She pauses for a moment. "Looking at these quotes involves revisiting places we've been," she says. "Some of those places were hard places, hard for the group, hard for each one of us, in different ways. Just so you're alert to that, as you start moving along the walls." A few people nod. "Okay," she says. "Let's go."

Then we are crowded at one end of the brightly lit corridor. People jockey a bit for position, so they can see the quotes properly. And then the hall goes quiet.

Excerpts from *What it took for the group: What happened and what needed to happen, for this drama to be created*

"At the beginning, we didn't really have an under-standing of metastatic cancer—we didn't understand what they were suffering."

"After Ross read the statistics there was a sort of hush over the group for just a second and I kinda looked around and I thought, okay, we've said it now, now let's pass it, because it can't be what governs us."

"In the early stages there was the real 'not knowing' around the illness issues, and then having to apply that to these real women who are sitting there and to dance with that. The move forward but the move back, almost the dangerousness of it in a way."

"We had to find a key of under-standing that all people could partake in."

"I really respected the actors' willingness to put themselves into a potentially painful situation, or at least anxiety producing."

"Part of the journey was beginning to understand that Jan and Mary Sue were far more than just their disease. But that couldn't happen until we actually began to get to know each other."

"Everybody here has had some tragedy. Metastatic disease is just one of many things that are happening. The rest of you have stories to be told as well. I think it's a matter of getting to know people as much as any-thing, what they're like and how they are. Them knowing me, and me knowing them as well."

"If you don't have that particular experience of metastatic breast cancer, then you link it to other things. I think people began to get the idea that there are related experiences in life that put you into that space where you don't know what is going to happen next and where you are."

"Everyone is looking for a structure and it's knowing that this is a wide structure: let people flounder for a little while."

"We use what the other people have said in the focus groups to say, 'what does this mean to me?' And then we go back into ourselves and bring out our own associations and relationships to that."

"I realized that night when I was hashing through it that my hope was totally hinged on a cure for Mary Sue and Jan and everybody else. Suddenly there was this denial, not denial of their experience or what they are going through, but a really strong fervent resistance to death. To their deaths... But with that also a real understanding of some of the anguish and the fear and the hope and the everything that they and their families and friends must go through because at that point I was living it as well, and I know I was not the only one."

"The project required us to truly understand what was going on with metastatic disease, but also I think it had to sink in what it meant to us individually. I think we got onto an emotional level with it as well, and I think only when we hit that level were we really ready to work on the project."

"These groups—people who are well, and people who had been sick but are now well, and then people who are not well—found their way to some common ground. Everybody moving into the space occupied by the ill women, and taking that up, being willing to take that up."

"Don't tell anybody this. The panic and the fear of not feeling there's a product looming is really important."

"I'm glad we took the risk that we might hurt people."

"Progressively people from the Sunnybrook side as it were, opened to the understanding of the illness from the people in the theater... Like it's a cross fertilization, the theater people showed understanding and fresh insights around the illness and the Sunnybrook people showed fresh insights about the theater so it was a marvelous crossover."

It is silent for a long time. People move slowly along the wall, pausing, reading the words, remembering.

When we gather in the room, Vrenia is crying, her hand over her mouth. Mary Sue crosses the room, puts her head on Vrenia's shoulder, cries with her. In the back of the room, Ann takes Jan's hand across the aisle.

"It was quite a thing, wasn't it," Christina says quietly. "Quite a thing." There is silence for a moment. "Does anyone . . . " she pauses, trying to tread gently "want to talk about reading those quotes? Tell us about your responses to them?"

Patricia speaks first. "It all comes back to me now. It brings the reality back into focus again. I think we've had so much fun doing it that we've forgotten about all the bad feelings at the beginning. The scary feelings."

"I think you've got it up there," Sandy says, gesturing to the hallway. "Because it's frightening to read it again."

"So something must be right," Christina says, "because it was frightening at the time?"

"Yeah, absolutely."

"It's sobering," someone says.

Mary Sue blows her nose, joins the conversation. "I think it's quite amazing," she says, "because, I mean, I've heard those quotes, I've been through the process, but . . . I think, as Patricia said, when we play, it's just been such a wonderful experience, sometimes I forget what it is that we're doing."

She hesitates, then adds, "Except that we're stars!" Smiles break out around the room. We're all delighted with Mary Sue's newfound "diva" status.

"For me," says Jan, "this group has been an extended support group, like a group of cheerleaders. The demons never go away. But so many people care."

"The demons are there for us too, in regards to you two," Vrenia says, looking up at Jan, distress in her voice. "And I'd forgotten. I'd forgotten." She pauses a moment. "Talk about denial," she says wryly.

"It works," says Mary Sue. "Denial and scotch."

"Chinese food and beer," Jan says.

Again, there is silence. "I think what strikes me too when I read that," Jan says slowly, "is that there's almost an innocence. There's a . . . "

"I'd call it cluelessness," Ross interjects.

Everyone laughs, then Jan carries on. "There's the feeling of discovery, like in the improvs, to feel that we've touched that piece of information, we've given life to that quote from the transcripts. The wonder of being part of it, being involved."

"At the beginning," Patricia says, "you think, 'Are they crazy? How are they going to make a play out of all this?' And it just seemed to unfold and unfold. It was really incredible, the whole process."

"Another thing for me, at this point in time," says Vrenia, "is the feeling of not being able to take in the impact that the drama is having on others. There's not a nerve or a gene in me that helps me process that. The best we can do is poke fun at it. I always quote Ross on this: 'We were wonderful, people said we changed their lives—you know, the usual.'"

People chuckle, and then Vrenia continues. "I know how it feels, but I can't even voice what it does to me. That doctors go and talk about the emotional impact of treating people with cancer, or with terminal illness. I mean, that's amazing. That people thank us, that people cry, that people say, 'I needed this'—all those responses. And the corollary of that, because that's happened, the love I feel for people in this room increases. I mean, thank you," she says, looking around the room "thanks for all of us doing this."

Murmurs of agreement around the room. "Thank you," says Christina. "That's great. Does anyone have anything else to add to the quotes?"

"I think for me what was missing was something about the laughter," says Jan. "It wasn't there at the beginning, but it became so much a part of what we did. I remember—not to pick on Lou—but when he stood up that first time we were rehearsing and instead of saying, 'the ten best offers of help,' he stood up straight and tall and said it out: 'the ten *breast* offers of help . . .'"

Everyone laughs, recalling it. "And we all lost it," Jan continues. "I mean, we were hysterical, and he was looking at us, I don't think he realized what he'd said. The tears, the laughing. The laughter became as important as the tears, as the understanding, the fears."

We talk more about laughter, about how it was nervous at first, or hiding something, and about the moment when it became the kind of laughter that bubbles among us now. "There was a period of time when we couldn't get through a rehearsal without crazy things happening," Vrenia says. "It was usually Mrs. Vanstone there"—she looks over at Elaine—"who got the ball rolling."

Marg smiles broadly. "I was just remembering the Thunder Bay trip, when I was the prompter. The rehearsal was moving along. Then you got to the support group scene. And I could see this grin starting on Mary Sue's face, and little giggle. And she got to those lines. . . ."

"Overwhelmed by Family" from the *Handle with Care?* Script

I am the glue. I feel that I am holding things together. And my husband seems to be going through something like—as though this was, like, his problem more than mine. And I almost feel that he needs more help, maybe more attention, than I do. I feel like, at this point, that I am stronger. And he needs to be stroked. I mean, the man has no health problems to speak of. Why does he need to be stroked?

"You got to the line about your husband being stroked," says Marg, "and you all just fell apart."

Howls of laughter fill the room. "That was Elaine," someone exclaims. "She started that."

"Every time I see the play now, I hold my breath when you get to that part," Marg says, still chuckling about it.

"Me too," says Patricia.

"We all hold our breath," Vrenia says.

Mary Sue leans forward, intense. "The energy that we all derive from doing this," she says, gesturing around the room. "I know there were days when I dragged my ass to get down there to Ryerson. And I'd come out feeling better after working hard on it. It is energizing. I don't know what it is, but I have felt it."

"There's not too many things I'd take a 7:30 A.M. bus for," says Jan, referring to her two-hour trek from Orillia to Toronto for all of our rehearsals.

We shift into talking about how people feel more able to connect with friends and family who are ill or suffering because of their participation in the project. And then Vrenia asks, "Can I share some really painful things?"

Everyone nods, and the tone shifts with the strain and sadness in her voice. "Once the script was written, it was the five parts. And suddenly Mary Sue gets hit with the line, 'I'm going to die.' There were some really difficult moments there, in some of the lines that came out."

"Yes," says Christina. "And in who they landed with, and when."

"Yeah," says Vrenia, nodding. "Because there's almost a little warrior that goes, 'Okay, nothing is going to happen. It's all going to be good, right?' And to a certain extent, the laughter plays into that. I sort of feel that if we can just keep laughing, that the demons will stay away. What is it that you get when you laugh?"

"Endorphins," someone says.

"The endorphins will keep all cancer cells at bay, right, so if we can just"—she speaks each word carefully—"keep laughing. We loved the laughter, it made us feel good and healthy but it also has a much stronger . . . "

"It was connected to the unfunny pieces," says Ann.

"The laughter was," Vrenia pauses, chooses her statement, "absolutely necessary. To save us, from whatever might be lurking."

It is almost time for us to end the meeting. "Let's finish off with some discussion about what we learned in creating *Handle with Care?*" Christina says. "If twelve people walked into this room who wanted to do a research-based theater project and we had"—she looks at her watch—"twenty minutes with them, what would you tell them?"

"Never say never," Patricia says.

"I would immediately start them on their feet," says Vrenia.

We head off on some tangent, and Christina poses her question another way. "Is there anything we should have done differently?" she asks.

"Differently, how?" Vrenia wants to know. "To move us along faster?"

"To spare us pain?" Ann asks, almost at the same moment, with the slightest hint of irony in her voice.

"Well," says Christina, "there was a lot of anxiety and concern at the beginning of the process . . . "

Marg joins in, talking about her experience leading palliative care workshops. "When people are anxious at these workshops, I don't get distressed," she says. "I know where the outcome is going to come. Here, there were no frames of reference for me, no signposts. I didn't therefore have the ability to keep my own anxiety in check."

"In terms of working on the prostate cancer show now," Ross says, "there's lots of anxiety. Will the script be good? Will we find the right actors? But I'm not anxious in the same way as I was before because I know that there are about five signposts that I'll recognize."

Vrenia raises her eyebrows at him. "Oh, really? Will you let me know what they are?"

"Well, you know, we'll reach the end of the script, and then we'll have rehearsals—oh, okay!" Ross replies, "I can see that now."

"But the anxiety is before you get to that point," counters Vrenia.

"Yes, and I'm not talking about taking all that anxiety out, but knowing that there are several predictable things that you move through," says Ross. "And in *Handle with Care?* I really had no idea what those were. And like Marg, that really . . . " Ross stretches back into his chair, throwing his arms out to convey the weight of living for so long with the uncertainty of the creative process and what, if anything, might emerge from it.

Vrenia laughs. "I could feel the fear radiating from you," she says to him. She turns to Christina. "My experience with these shows is that ultimately, it comes together. You know, in *Shakespeare in Love*—'It's a mystery.' And something happens. It does happen."

"But you've seen it happen," Marg protests. "You've had the past experience of seeing it happen. But for those of us who are new to that particular experience, we didn't have that."

"That was good, though," Vrenia says passionately.

"It's a necessary part of the project, I think, to be out there with no safety net," Dvora affirms. Dvora is a member of Act II Studio, and she wrote the "Magda the magician" scene in *Handle with Care?*—the scene that Mary Sue used to enact the diva in herself.

Christina wants to talk about another source of anxiety early in the project. "Some of the people I interviewed said they would have appreciated more information about metastatic disease up front. And there were two pieces to that: the facts, and what the emotional engagement with that knowledge can mean. Other people I talked to said, 'That part can't be rushed. You have to let that process unfold.'"

Mary Sue looks doubtful. "If people heard it the first day, could they take it in?"

"I remember when Marg presented this stuff to us," Sandy says. "We did get it, but it was hard to receive at first."

"It's like having a baby and someone telling you what it's going to be like," Mary Sue says. "You don't believe them anyway. You have to experience it."

"You can also scare people off," says Ross. "And I think that having done this kind of project once, you can draw on the range of experiences that people have. For a new group, that would be a great way of getting informed consent. You can say, 'We did a project about cancer before. Some of the people had trouble sleeping at night, some people went through some tough times in this way and that way, and most of the people felt that it was really worth it in the end, but not everybody, and you need to know that.'"

"If everybody had come into those first two meetings and was told exactly what metastatic breast cancer was," said Mary Sue, "I'm not sure anybody would have come back. It wouldn't have given us a chance to talk about our feelings about it. And the vulnerability that Patricia talked about early on made me really aware of where other people were at. I think that was as important a part of the process as the creative part."

"I think there's a real value in the naiveté, in learning as you go," says Jan. "If you gave me one sentence, I would say to this group: Don't rush it. You don't rush your research. You're methodical, you organize it, you labor over it, you make it make the best sense you can. Do that with your theater. Don't try to push people through the steps because they need to crawl before they walk."

"I would say, Hire Vrenia," says Dvora.

"Are you kidding?" Elaine looks affronted. "You have to take all of us."

Everyone laughs, and applauds, and amidst a flurry of hugs, we disperse.

❋

It wasn't our intention, at that meeting in June, to reach a consensus about the virtues or vices of panic in a creative process. Though most people concurred that a certain "letting go" was required—a willingness to follow paths that might be uncomfortable or appear unproductive, to open and reopen ideas, struggles, scenes—in the final analysis, we still held conflicting beliefs about just how much free fall (and attendant panic) was necessary.

In the interviews Christina conducted over the course of the drama's development, some people clearly had been distressed at what they perceived as insufficient preparation for the *Handle with Care?* journey. A few were dismayed at the apparent lack of structure for our work together, or angry about our early floundering in relation to the illness issues. Others, of course, felt that floundering was an absolutely essential component of our task.

In a way, this ethical debate about how carefully people should or can be "held" in such a project, and the level of uncertainty one has to embrace in it all, resonates with the question mark in the drama's title. "Handle with Care" surfaces common responses to people living with serious illness: often we approach them as if they are dangerous, unpredictable, to be wary of; or, as if they are fragile, vulnerable, needing protection. So, too, with this project: at different times, various people perceived it as dangerous, or perceived people involved in it as requiring something more or different than they were getting—more information, more attention to the emotional toll, more assurance about the path we were on and the outcomes we might anticipate.

And while it seemed important to review people's concerns and convictions about how the project unfolded, it's difficult to imagine what we might offer to others out of this process. Take two parts less angst and chaos, add a modicum more of information, and you'll have it just right? A recipe some of us might endorse, but a hell of a thing to actually bake.

Researcher Rant: September 2000: Ross

I am on the phone to our publisher, Mitch Allen, talking about issues related to the videotape that accompanies this manuscript. As the conversation is winding down, he turns to another topic. He hopes we are planning to discuss our second dramatic production, *No Big Deal?* in some detail in our writing, and that we will compare our experiences in that project with *Handle with Care?* He reasserts a position we have heard before, that such comparisons will help readers to understand the principles of our work, to see the larger picture beyond the details of one story, one project. I mumble something intended to placate Mitch for the moment and get off the phone.

Shortly after that conversation, I sent Christina an email message saying that we needed to talk again about what to do with *No Big Deal?* Clearly, our argument that we wanted to tell a single story, not two, had only been partially successful. And maybe there would indeed be benefit, I wrote, in trying to weave in the *No Big Deal?* stuff—if we could manage to do it in a way that didn't suggest there was a straightforward formula for this kind of work, in a way that honored our group's warning to not provide too much guidance, too much structure to others interested in research-based theater. Like qualitative researchers everywhere, we were treading that difficult ground between valuing the specifics of each separate experience in its own right and hoping that the learning from one experience can have relevance for another. We decided we would do our best to let the two projects illuminate each other, while at the same time advocating for flexibility with this type of work, and taking the position that each new project has to be approached in terms of its own unique characteristics.

Part of what distinguished the development of *No Big Deal?* from that of *Handle with Care?* was that I now had a sense of the steps that would have to be taken to produce a script and its enactment. Although there was still plenty of room to worry, I was much more relaxed and able to enjoy myself. A particularly delicious moment occurred when Vrenia became upset with me for not taking the task seriously enough. In the midst of reviewing our draft script, she became suddenly concerned and asked me whether a particular scene was staying true to the original research transcripts. "Who cares? I like it," I replied. Vrenia looked at me with astonishment, bordering on panic. This was not the response she had come to count on. She was used to holding down the creative playfulness end of the continuum, knowing she could count on me to hold down the other end, to keep asking whether we were connected closely enough with the experiences of the people we interviewed in our studies. But I was now ready to take more risks in the writing, ready to trust my dramatic interpretations instead of constantly deferring to the word-for-word transcripts. While I was still concerned to reflect the perspectives of the men and women in our original study, my focus now was more with the meanings that were at play than the words themselves.

In the long run, our script maintained a solid link to the spoken words of couples we interviewed, but there was a great deal of playful experimentation with interpretative scenes along the way—some of which found their way into the production. One of my contributions in this regard was the character of "Professor Joker," a madcap professor who expounds about this and that and in the process reveals the crazy-making world into which men diagnosed with prostate cancer find themselves parachuted. Below is his first monologue, in which he introduces the audience to gendered aspects of illness.

D (PROFESSOR JOKER) [INTERRUPTING A]: Excuse me, sorry I'm late. This is the prostate cancer forum? Right? Thanks for holding down the fort. You can go now. Go! As you all know, I'm Professor Joker [LEADS AUDIENCE IN CLAPPING]

Now, the first point I wish to make is that when a man gets sick, it's a challenge for the space program. As you are all aware, and I must say that my own work has been critical to this matter, science has now firmly established that women are from Venus and men are from Mars. Those of you in a relationship know that communication between men and women can be a tad trying at the best of times. Throw in a man who is ill and it's suddenly more like men and women are from different universes. So scientists need to be working on ways for men and women to travel back and forth across these huge distances.

The saving grace is that we're talking about men here. I mean, if it was women who were ill, well, then we'd have to worry about serious distress, you know, weeping and wailing and that kind of thing. But my research into the emotional lives of men shows that men are more similar to slabs of granite than they are to women. There's this ridiculous idea, promoted by a group of female scientists in the U.S., that men are just repressing stuff like fear of death, grief about aging, and so on, but my team is on the verge of proving, once and for all, that for men, it's really all NO BIG DEAL! [EXITS]

—From the *Handle with Care?* script

Vrenia had a flash of brilliance that led to another series of interpretive scenes that we scattered throughout the production, including the opening scene. The setting for these scenes is a battlefield, reflecting the language and images of war used by many of the men with prostate cancer we interviewed. As the drama begins, a man and a woman wearing army helmets weave and duck as they make their way to center stage amid the sounds of bombs exploding, and the clatter of machine-gun fire all around them. The man stops, looks at the woman. "So this is it. Time for battle." The woman glances at him, sidestepping a bullet, "I guess there's nothing for it. We'll do our best." The man starts to talk about the need to keep casualties to a minimum, about how they'll someday look back on this and laugh. In turn, the woman reassures the man that they're a fighting team, that all they have to do is stay positive. Suddenly a huge bomb explodes and the couple flees the stage in panic.

We had planned, in creating *No Big Deal?* to use *Handle with Care?* as a template. Our script development group would once again be comprised of researchers, volunteer actors, and individuals who had experienced cancer. But it proved much harder to put together a group for the new project. Older male actors were harder to find than women had been, as were men with prostate cancer who would be willing to participate in a theater project. I made an invitation to a huge room full of men at the local Man-to-Man prostate support group meeting, and only one expressed interest in participating.

Eventually, we found three prostate cancer patients willing to help, along with one man with another kind of cancer, and several women, mostly from Act II. Building on our discussions with the *Handle with Care?* crew, we took a more formal approach to getting "informed consent" from the *No Big Deal?* group members. We were explicit about how participation in the process could be distressing at times; we discussed possibilities for dealing with issues that might arise.

At the first meeting, the women outnumbered the men, a situation that continued throughout and eventually caused difficulties. None of the men with cancer were able to attend meetings regularly, creating a scattergun effect for their input. The women in the group out-talked the men, making it a constant challenge to make sure that the men's perspective was being properly included.

One obvious principle for a script development process is that sufficient constituents of each subgroup (researchers, actors, patients) must be present. This way, each can make a substantive contribution, and the group itself can reflect a range of perspectives. Things can get particularly thrown off if there is only one representative of a group and s/he speaks strongly from an extreme position. This happened at times in the *No Big Deal?* project, where, for example, one man with prostate cancer was adamant that any patients who denied being traumatized by post-treatment impotence were liars.

In looking back over both projects, we would also encourage others engaged in this work to be alert to the ways the broad social features of a health problem may surface within a script development group. In *Handle with Care?* it was the reluctance to go beyond a positive-thinking discourse when considering metastatic breast cancer. In *No Big Deal?* with its focus on couples, it was the strongly held biases about gender that men and women carried into the project. In both projects, we were insufficiently prepared for these factors, and in the *No Big Deal?* script development group, we never really got beyond the stereotypical beliefs of individual group members about what men were like, what women were like, and who was to blame for everything. In the end, Vrenia and I agreed to shorten the group process, deciding that it could not assist us further in establishing a foundation for the script.

Although we were less successful with our group work in *No Big Deal?* than we had been in the breast cancer project, we were able to make up for lost ground through a more intensive scriptwriting process. Vrenia and I spent a lot of time together hashing out and then rehashing various scenes, so that by the time we had a draft script, we felt we had accomplished everything that might have been accomplished through a broader group effort. But, wanting to be sure, we embarked on a more far-reaching feedback process (other readers and trial audiences of prostate cancer patients, health professionals, and theater people) than we had pursued with *Handle with Care?* In the end, despite their very different courses, both projects allowed for multiple perspectives and extensive input.

In *No Big Deal?* it turned out that I was the only individual who had participated both in the script development group and as an actor in the original cast. This is in marked contrast to *Handle with Care?* where all the original cast members had also been part of the script development process. While this meant that *No Big Deal?* actors had to learn about prostate cancer as they were also learning their acting lines, we have been very gratified by the strong commitment that cast members have made to the show. The opportunity to participate in a production that might benefit others seems to be highly motivating to older actors no longer on a track to try and achieve fame.

Another difference between the two projects is that no prostate cancer patients act in *No Big Deal?* While this does not allow for the extra poignancy that Mary Sue and Jan bring to *Handle with Care?* our experience has shown that there is still plenty of poignancy when actors commit themselves to agreed-upon representations of illness-related issues. Rather than a necessity, actors who represent the community under study are an added benefit.

When we first applied for funding for our research study about men with prostate cancer and their spouses, we described the likely outcome of our study to be a group information/ support intervention that would target couples. As we proceeded with interviews, it became increasingly apparent that a group intervention such as we had envisioned simply would not work. It seemed unlikely that any of the thirty-four men we spoke with, and very few of the women, would be interested or willing to be part of such an intervention. Whatever need our study participants might have had for information from other patients or spouses could already be met through existing prostate cancer self-help groups. And support was not something they (especially the men) were looking for outside of their marriages or other existing relationships.

We eventually substituted the idea of the drama for the structured group intervention. In the theater format, we argued to ourselves, couples could learn about issues without being forced into becoming active participants in discussion, without having to reveal their vulnerabilities and fears. But still, we wondered how older men would respond to the drama. Would they attend performances or stay at home and watch hockey instead? If they did attend, would they be open to dramatic representations of the prostate cancer experience? Would they participate meaningfully in postperformance discussions, or simply ask factual questions about the value of this treatment versus that treatment? We wondered if research-based theater was a heavily gendered phenomenon, with limited value for men, especially older men.

I was absolutely thrilled by our preview performance of *No Big Deal?* in Oshawa, a city just outside of Toronto, a key site for Canada's auto manufacturing industry. There were about 120 people in the audience, most of them men with prostate cancer and their wives. Throughout the performance, there was a lot of laughter and the occasional gasp. I could feel from the warmth of their response that we had gotten things right.

The discussion afterwards was remarkable. One man talked about the humor in the performance, saying "I've had prostate cancer for five years and tonight is the first time I've enjoyed it." His comment was greeted by a roar of laughter from others in the audience.

Another man asked if we'd be coming back to give a second performance. I said no, but there would be other performances in Toronto and elsewhere. He was glad to hear that, commenting, "I think my wife should see this. We've been married forty-five years but I haven't talked to her about my prostate cancer. I think it's time I did."

A forty-something woman in the front row put up a hand, the other hand still intertwined with her husband's. "You know, we've been dealing with all these issues for eight years now, but always on our own, in private. It's so amazing to see the same problems being presented in public. You don't feel so alone."

"Yes," I concurred, "prostate cancer has been pretty much hidden from public view until recently. And many of the couples I've talked with feel quite isolated with their struggles."

Interspersed with these comments were questions I couldn't answer about medical issues, and general expressions of pleasure about the play. When I sensed that the discussion was winding down, I called for one last comment or question.

A deep voice boomed out from the back, "I found this a very enjoyable evening. But more than that, I think it will help a lot of the couples here. I suspect there will be some interesting conversations over kitchen tables later tonight." The crowd murmured its approval. What more could we ask for by way of audience response?

So, while aspects of audience response to *No Big Deal?* (and *Handle with Care?*) are indisputably gendered, we now see the overall potential for research-based theater as being just as substantial for men as it is for women. Below are a few of the comments written on feedback forms from our six preview performances.

My husband and I have found our sense of humour has been one of our greatest strengths through this unfunny time. Thanks for the humorous part of your performance. (Spouse)

I wish this had been available for me to see after my surgery. I enjoyed the production throughout, but especially the parts about the relationship between man and wife. (Patient)

This is a wonderful method for sharing research with a wide audience. More "battle of the sexes" scenes than *I Love Lucy*. You've touched the audience. Well done. (Men's health scholar)

Very helpful to me should my day for prostate cancer come. The performance was superb. (Friend of prostate cancer patient)

This play has a strong emotional impact. I was very moved. Congratulations. (Physician)

It was useful to see the women's reactions. Even though we've been through it all, including impotence, I still learned more. (Patient)

It dispelled the myth that I had believed about prostate cancer being less serious. I also learned about what kinds of questions to ask. Very informative. (Medical resident)

While I am writing this, we are in the process of preparing to begin the official "tour" of *No Big Deal?* having completed a series of preview performances last spring. Our plan is to do fewer performances than we did for *Handle with Care?* although there probably would be sufficient interest to do at least as many. Instead of a run of two and a half years, we will perform for ten months and then close the show. While this plan makes enormous sense from time, energy, and financial perspectives, it will be sure to leave many men in communities across Canada disappointed. So we are going to rely more on videotape.

The first videotape version we made of *Handle with Care?* (not the one that's part of this package) the actors hated; I did too. It was adequate as a teaching tool, but not as a demonstration of the drama. We saw it as complementary, but never as a substitute for live performance.

Newly caught up in the excitement of theater, I was also quick to dismiss a colleague's suggestion that our approach was inefficient, that video and Internet showings of the play would make our work more accessible than the logistically complicated and relatively expensive live performances.

I am still strongly attached to the compelling quality of live drama. But for *No Big Deal?* I will travel to some cities on my own, show the filmed version, and facilitate a postscreening discussion similar to what we do after live performances. Like so much of our experience in *Handle with Care?* and *No Big Deal?* I don't know whether or how this will work. I don't know how effectively other forms of representation will reflect or evoke the experience of living with illness. But I find myself more and more willing to ask the question.

Researcher Rant: September 2000: Christina

From many standpoints, both *Handle with Care?* and *No Big Deal?* brought together—and eventually harmonized—a choir of voices. Many women's voices, and many men's voices, spoke through the dramas, and gender—beliefs about men and women, and gendered aspects of illness and support-giving—

often came to the fore. Still, many voices, and many social realities, were absent. Occasionally, audience members remarked on those absences. A woman who had seen *Handle with Care?* noted that the particular struggles faced by young women with metastatic breast cancer—how hard it is to talk with small children about the illness, for instance—went unspoken. Others asked about, or commented on, the specific challenges faced by Aboriginal women, Chinese women, and women whose first language is not English. More than one man who saw *No Big Deal?* asked why the drama had not addressed issues of advanced hormone-refractory disease or bone pain.

When these absences were made visible after a performance, we sometimes referred back to the original studies. Each drama presented the experiences of people in the situations and circumstances of those who had participated in the research. In the study about metastatic breast cancer, none of the women were Chinese or Aboriginal. And while they were, on average, eight years younger than the average Canadian woman with breast cancer, most were over forty. The prostate cancer study involved men in the first year posttreatment, so none of them were in the kinds of difficulties audience members sometimes described.

In most research contexts, it is legitimate to say, "These were the limitations of this study, this was the sample, this leaves us unable to comment on such and such." Then you're off the hook, more or less. But in a public setting, a "limitation" of the study—understood by many researchers as a relatively neutral boundary, a parameter, a delineation—becomes a shortcoming. Here, the issue of who gets included is less about justifying a sampling frame and more about responding to people's experiences and life circumstances, responding to people who are asking, "What about my story?"

At the meeting in June 1999 when we discussed the introduction of new actors, we also had a conversation—a fairly brief conversation, sandwiched in between all the other activities of that day—about the experiences that were missing from *Handle with Care?* Jan commented that there was nothing in the drama that spoke to the specific challenges faced by single women with metastatic disease. "I envy people with partners," she said. "I've had to struggle with this illness alone, especially at night."

"Perfect," someone said. "Let's use that." And Vrenia went to work writing Jan's words into the opening scene.

I remember being quite grumpy at that moment. Not about Jan's line making it in, of course. I had already substituted the word "partner" for "husband" in another scene, in a gesture—very small, but a gesture nonetheless—to the lesbians in the audience, and to heterosexual couples for whom the terms "husband" and "wife" don't fit. What I was grumpy about was the seeming arbitrariness with which some voices were added to the mix and others were not. People felt that any attention to ethnic and cultural diversity, for instance, would require an entirely new research undertaking.

In a way, this response did point to the origin of the problem. The original research was both a foundation of strength for the drama, and the source of its limitations.

In a subsequent project, Ross has expanded the scope of study with men with prostate cancer. He and his team have been collecting life histories of gay and African Canadian men with prostate cancer, looking at how illness fits within the context of their lives and their constructions of masculinity. This study could eventually bring different stories to the stage. Like the gay man who told Ross that it's more difficult to come out of the closet about prostate cancer than it was about sexual preference. Or the black man who used his experience with illness to lever stronger input of cultural minorities into health programs in his workplace.

More and more varied voices can be made audible, then, in other kinds of research processes. In the last several months, we have also thought about, and come across in other people's writing (Gingrich-Philbrook 1998; Park-Fuller 2000), ways to address absent voices in the context of the performance itself, and in the postperformance discussion. When someone who has seen *No Big Deal?* asks why none of the men in the drama have advanced prostate cancer, Ross now makes a point of problematizing our decision to curtail the performance to match sampling parameters. Should the drama, in fact, deal only with issues and circumstances that arose or were present in the research? Or is too much left out? Here, then, the choices we made along the way about the drama's link to the research, and the choices made in the research process itself, are offered up for debate.

Park-Fuller (2000), writing about staged personal narratives, suggests other strategies. In her performance about breast cancer, a timer sounds every twelve minutes, to symbolize the frequency with which people die of breast cancer in the United States. She claims that this device calls audience attention to the fact that so many women's voices are absent from her testimony, and gives people the power to contradict her story.

She also points us to a renewed understanding of audience responses to the performance. While we have taken people's comments about absent voices as critique (and, of course, they have occasionally been intended as such), Park-Fuller encourages us to perceive such comments as an integral and valued part of the drama, serving (at least) two purposes. Discussion following a performance is, on the one hand, a chance for the stories told in *Handle with Care?* and *No Big Deal?* to "listen . . . very carefully for the counsel of [their] kin" (Gingrich-Philbrook 1998 cited in Park-Fuller 2000, 33). Audience members' stories inform, and may well argue, with the performers' tale, and we all learn from a dialogue generated with the performance. On the other hand, in this framework, audience members' voices can be understood as part of the performance, a telling, in yet another voice, of the drama's story.

✻

CHAPTER NINE

TRAVELING, UNRAVELING

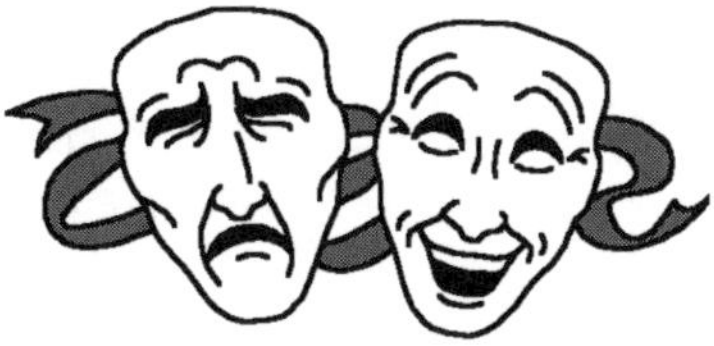

In September 1999, we embark on the second leg of our Ontario tour. The schedule Fran draws up has us performing nineteen times in September and October. On September 21, a troupe appears in Peterborough, in the central part of the province; three days later, another troupe flies out to Timmins, about 700 kilometers north. A week after that, on the same day, performances take place in Kingston and on Manitoulin Island.

And then we get word from the Canadian Breast Cancer Foundation: the national tour is a go. Fran becomes the center of a logistical storm, creating lists and sublists, making endless phone calls to hotels and travel agents.

Deciding who will go on what trip is an especially complex algorithm. The bags of props, despite their clever organization, are heavy and somewhat unwieldy; we need at least two people who can haul them up and down stairs, through airports, across parking lots. Someone in each crew will have to drive the rental van. We need at least one person who can facilitate the health professional performance, and one who's been with the production from the start, to answer questions about the history. Some venues seem to call out for Jan or Mary Sue to be there; others require Ross.

And, of course, we all want to go to certain parts of the country. Fran's answering machine fills up with messages from people who have cousins in Calgary, nieces in Nova Scotia, sons in Saskatoon, best friends in Banff. Or we want to travel with particular people from the cast. Or we can go only if we can return on an early flight, or a late flight, or the day after. To complicate matters even further, several cast members are involved in rehearsals for an upcoming Act II Studio production. A low-level tug of war starts for their time and attention.

And then, in January, Mary Sue receives the news from her oncologist: there are more tumors in her liver. She begins chemotherapy, again. Loses her hair, again. And we are grieving, again.

Memorybank Drama: February 2000, Robert Gill Theatre, Toronto: Christina

Tension slides around backstage. Mary Sue is lying on the bed, pale, nauseated. Struggling with diarrhea.

When they call us she sits up, gathers herself together. We walk out and take our places on the stage. The performance unfolds. We arrive at the "summer rant," a scene taken almost directly from one of the focus group transcripts. Mary Sue speaks it:

You're told, like, "Enjoy your summer," you know what I mean? He took me by the hand, and, you know what I mean. It doesn't take a rocket scientist to figure out what you're saying. Enjoy your summer because it's your last one. But at the same time, I was told "when this treatment stops working" . . . and I said to him, "When?" I said, "*If*, not when. Who are you to decide it's going to fail?"

It's like, "well, most treatments, the longest they'll last, depending on the type of chemotherapy, depending on the patient, will only work for so long." And it's fine to quote statistics, but at the same time, you don't know. And he also sat there and told me there are patients who have lived longer. And what if I'm one of them? And you're telling me—you know, if you plant a seed, it's there—I've got this set period of time. I didn't live because I was anticipating the end. And here I am a year later. And I know he has responsibilities as a physician. And I'm not asking to be given some kind of false hope. I'm fairly intelligent, and I don't expect that. But don't write me off!

—From the *Handle with Care?* script

The last line rings in my ears; the vehemence in her voice takes my breath away.

When the performance is over, we all sit at the front of the stage, receiving questions, offering comment. In the back, a young woman with a scarf on her head raises her hand. Her words are full with emotion. "I can't tell you how you ladies have touched my soul this evening. You are so special," she says. She looks directly at Mary Sue and Jan, pauses, and grins. "And you are so—cool!"

"Cool" is utterly unexpected, and utterly perfect. Mary Sue throws her head back, laughing and clapping. Jan's pleasure beams around the room. I am delighted by this woman, and so relieved to feel myself relaxing into enjoyment again.

Then a woman in the front row puts up her hand. I had noticed her earlier, registered her unsmilingness. The facilitator invites her to speak. Her voice is measured. "You don't talk about death in this play. Was this a deliberate decision?"

The whole room stills. Anxiety ricochets through my body. No, I think. No, don't do this.

We look at each other, stutter a bit. Jan picks it up. "We made a decision to focus on hope," she says. "The women in the research really wanted to talk about living *with* this disease."

"Yet death is everywhere," Ross protests. "It underlies every moment in the drama."

I am silent. She is angry, I think. She or someone she loves is living—or more likely dying—with this disease. And we have not told her story. I feel we have abandoned her. I feel abandoned myself. Suddenly, none of it is enough. Not for this woman. Not for me, for what I have felt this evening, watching Mary Sue in that bed. It is not enough. We are not enough.

Memorybank Drama: June 1999: Ross

The decisions Vrenia and I made about how many people to have available for each role in the drama were logistical and practical, and a lot else besides. We had agreed that the ideal number was three. That would allow for one official back-up for each role for every performance and would also mean there were some performances people wouldn't have to be available for at all, either as actors or back-ups.

I'd been worried about asking too much of the cast, especially the people from Act II Studio. But it soon became clear that nobody was worried about doing too much acting—quite the opposite: practically everyone was worried they wouldn't get enough opportunities on the stage.

This was especially difficult to sort out with Mary Sue and Jan, who were in a somewhat different category from everyone else. We all agreed that when one or both of them were part of the cast, it added an extra dimension to performances. And we wanted to give them every opportunity we could. But we also wanted to be fair to the other cast members, who had spent so many hours in rehearsal. Vrenia and I spent a lot of time talking and negotiating about this.

Just before the meeting where Christina presented the information she'd been gathering through interviews with the script development group, I learned that Mary Sue was due to start treatment again. I remembered how difficult it was for her during her last bout of chemotherapy. I was virtually certain that this new round of treatment would lead, at best, to a disruption of her availability for acting. At worst, with the treatment signaling progression of disease, she could become actively ill; she might need to be hospitalized. We could lose her entirely from the cast.

Then there was Phyllis and Elaine, the other women who played the same role as Mary Sue (the 'C' role). Phyllis missed several months of performances during the winter because of problems related to her own health. Would she be well enough to act? And Elaine has a chronically bad back. Her capacity to endure the rigors of touring with *Handle with Care?* seemed tenuous.

I phoned Vrenia, making the case that we needed another woman to be available to play the C role. She agreed, somewhat reluctantly, and volunteered to call Gloria about learning the part.

Soon after that, I started to hear the rumblings, brought to me second- and third-hand, about the unhappiness of the three women playing the C role. After the June meeting, where we introduced Gloria to the rest of the cast, Jan told me how upset Mary Sue was that we were adding a fourth person. No other role would have that many actors assigned to it. Were we giving up on her? Did we think she was dying?

I phoned Vrenia and we shared our anguish at having caused Mary Sue this harm. We decided to change the plan, ask Gloria to step down. If we needed another actor later, we'd make it happen then. We would support Mary Sue, carry on as if she were perfectly healthy. Gloria was understanding when we told her; Mary Sue was ecstatic.

Later, I apologized to Mary Sue, explaining my worries related to treatment effects. She scolded me, saying that we could count on her to be there to the end of the performances. She also told me that her oncologist had said that she should still be okay by next summer. That surprised me. Good news, I thought. And the lesson, again, straight from the script: don't write me off.

❃

The national tour—about thirty-five performances—ran from March until May. Here are some of the moments we remember best.

From Elaine

My first trip was to Yellowknife and there were many exciting things about that. First of all, there was dear Fran getting a van and starting off into the tundra with the rest of us. She hadn't had a lot of experience driving a van but you wouldn't know it if she hadn't told you.

Before we went, I asked, because I'm interested in details, how we were being transported because of the props and everything, and Ross said, "We're going to get a van." So that was fine. And then, when I looked at the list, I checked to see who might be drivers, and it wasn't obvious. So I called Fran and said, "Who's going to drive?" She said, "I am." She said, "We're getting a van this weekend and I'm going to learn to drive it."

And you asked about my faith—I've got all kinds of it [laughing].

She did so well and this was really one of the highlights of that trip, which was long and we had to make transfers and so on, and Fran just looked after everything like a really professional manager. The van was there; we were where we were supposed to be; she had done the map research and drove it with "assistance" from everyone in the vehicle, and just kept her cool. Really kept her cool. There were times when, well, when a couple of us did comment, but not Fran. She just kept on going and smiling.

From Ross

About 400 people turned out for the community performance in St. John's, Newfoundland. Beforehand, there was a lot of milling, people chatting, sort of like everybody knew everybody. But it was not a cancer-focused audience. They were just people. And that was rare. It became a community event. You felt like you had stepped into a larger context, and you were making a unique contribution to the community.

From Mary Sue

The best moments in the national tour were in some ways the same as they've been everywhere: the giggling and laughing in rehearsal. It was so wonderful.

We'd often go to some little bar that someone would find. And at odd times, because you'd have an afternoon show and an evening show, so you were out at 3:00 in the afternoon at some pub, where only the drunks, or nobody else, is there. And you're tired, but you're wound up. Those were fun times.

It reminded me of some of the early trips in Ontario. Now that was early on, so we were going to party. We were still talking about going dancing. Right [laughs]. And I remember once we went to an Irish bar, and some of us had fish and chips and beer, and we were all sort of hyper. And you could just watch us all sort of going like this [she wilts into the chair] saying, "Oh, dear, it's time to go to bed. We'll do the dancing some other time." There was always the promise of partying, which never really happened [laughs].

From Elaine

Did you hear about the lemon pie experience? There was a gift shop that we were all drawn to, and five of us were in it the afternoon of the community performance. And people were buying, people were looking, people were talking. We all ended up at the cash register while somebody paid for what they were getting. And the two shop ladies realized we were strangers, obviously, and so we told them why we were there. And oh, yes, they knew about the play. And were they going to come?

And so, Fran or Sandra, it may have been Sandra, said: "Well, bring ripe tomatoes because, you know, the green ones hurt. So bring ripe tomatoes to throw." And I said, "Well, if you don't have tomatoes, a lemon pie would be great. I'd far rather have a lemon pie thrown at me than tomatoes." This was about 4 o'clock and we went and changed and went to the hall. And just as I came in the door, everybody said: "Oh, Elaine, come, come, come." And I said "There's plenty of time," and anyway I got there and one of the ladies from the shop had gone home and made a lemon pie and was there with it. We decided not to have it bronzed. We ate it. We've got a picture of the lemon pie and the two ladies from the store, but you know, isn't that touching? And that is just so demonstrative of the flat-out way that we were welcomed.

From Patricia

Sometimes I could feel myself getting a little teary during some of the performances. And if I really start to think about Mary Sue and Jan and their situation, then I lose myself. You know. If I ever stop to think of them as the person, as the one that we're talking about, that this show is all about them. . . . That's what I couldn't let myself do when I was performing. A couple of times I did, I know, and I could feel my voice going. I remember one time Elaine said to me, "I thought you were going to lose it." And I said, "I thought I was going to lose it too."

From Elaine

When we went to the hospital in Yellowknife—it's a small hospital, obviously—and I suppose that thirty people maybe got into the room and we had about this much space [shows a small square of the room] to do the performance. But wonderful, wonderful feeling. They liked it so much that they wanted to get it to the three outposts, Fort Smith, and I forget the names of the other two. So we said, fine, we'll come back and do it. And so we did. We came back in a couple of hours and ran it again with the video hook-up. And that was just one of those little delightful things. They were so appreciative of us doing it twice. And, of course, we could hardly wait to do it twice.

And then we went to the community hall. And it got to be 7:25 P.M. and there were three people in the building. And that was including the two ladies with the lemon pie. And you know, we didn't want to say anything. Then one of the ladies said, "You're looking a bit anxious but you don't need to be. People don't come in Yellowknife until it's on time." And within seven minutes, they were putting extra chairs in. It was just as if a caribou herd had come in. The doors opened and they just appeared and it was full! And the response there, the questions, and there were full families there because somehow or another they had been alerted, you know, to bring people and again the atmosphere was wonderful and there was this reception after and they had home-baked everything.

From Ross

I didn't go on the early tours, but I took a lot of pleasure hearing the reports back—that people had such a good time in Yellowknife, for example. I got some flak for it, but I planned that one trip so it would be just Act II Studio people. I felt like they needed some time in the sun, all on their own, and I wanted them to have some opportunity doing it themselves. And people just really enjoyed that tour. I don't know that those two things were connected at all—it was partly just the

Yellowknife people, their response and so forth—but I was really pleased that it went so well.

From Jan

One of the things I remember very vividly is Vrenia's absolute delight at our accommodation in Victoria. We all had to go to everybody else's room, to see what they were like. She was just so excited. She was going off by herself to have tea at the Empress Hotel, and then Sandy decided to go with her. It's been a dream of Vrenia's forever, to have high tea at each of the CN (Canadian National) hotels. So off they went, the two of them, to spend forty-eight dollars to have tea. That was great.

From Mary Sue

One of the best things was playing to a big audience—not even a big audience, although that was fun—but playing to an appreciative audience.

I remember Fran was worried when she realized that Debbie Grant [executive director of the Canadian Breast Cancer Foundation's Atlantic Chapter] was going to be a kind of groupie, following us. Fran thought that might cramp our style. But what it meant was that Debbie had been to each place and she got people enthusiastic and organized about the drama. And she was there again, and they had a connection with her. It was so well done. You didn't realize how well it was done until you went somewhere else. Debbie was the front person, she made the difference. She really did.

So really I thought the Maritime tour was great. There were lots of people at each performance; it felt like we were anticipated, wanted, appreciated, people were excited about it. That made everybody feel good, so there wasn't that little bit of sniping that happened on some of the other tours.

From Ross

What I was worried about—and this was a common sticking point for me—was that we get good venues and good audiences. I worked for months trying to set up this performance at the Canadian Association of Psychosocial Oncology conference in Vancouver. And finally, we got the word that they were going to have us on the program. It was a bit complicated because there were two American associations and one Canadian association cohosting this, so the Canadians had to convince the Americans it was a good idea.

So once they had decided on it, I said, "We're really only interested if we perform in front of all of the delegates"—that's the new policy, right? They set us up for the first thing on the first day and then there was nothing else that day; the conference started mainly on the next morning. So I didn't know how many people we'd have. And they didn't know. They said maybe a third to a half of the delegates. So I was thinking, maybe we'll have a small audience. We'll do all of this work, and it will end up being not that satisfying.

But it was a pretty good audience, it was probably two-thirds of the delegates. And it was an audience that was right there from the get-go because they were all working in the field, they knew exactly what we were presenting, the sensitivities about it. I guess it was the closest to a group of peers that I'd ever presented to. And it was the usual enthusiastic response; we got a standing ovation and so forth. We got all kinds of invitations from that.

From Patricia

I remember giving you all your Qi.[1]. . . I worked at Wellesley Hospital about six years ago, and this doctor came there who was very involved in Qi. It's to pull yourself up, your energy; I can't say it like she can, but you're pulling all your energy "up."

And she was giving demonstrations. Well I thought, this is—you know—a crock. And then she picked me from the audience, to do it. And when she did it I truly believed it.

I'd forgotten all about this Qi thing, because it's years ago since I worked at Wellesley. But I must have been reading an article again on Qi, and I thought I would try it on you guys. I was hoping that I was giving you positive energy, because that's the theory of doing it, that I'm lifting your spirits, making you feel "I can do it." And there was that administrator at the hospital in Calgary who came along and said, "Could you give me some of that, then?" [laughs]

From Christina

I only went on one trip, the Alberta one. Lots of things stand out for me. I had a wonderful day with Dave, one of the newest troupe members, poking around the art galleries of Edmonton, and talking about *Handle with Care?* I really enjoyed being with Ross and his partner, Kathryn, in Red Deer and feeling like I had some small window into the kinds of communities in which the two of them grew up. And the performance in Calgary for health professionals was extraordinary. I was really moved by that.

But I guess what is most acutely with me from that trip is Jan's absence. She'd had that hellish week of radiation treatment early in March after they found the lesions on her skull. And then she rallied, and did the trips to Manitoba and British Columbia. I remember Elaine talking about her being kind of guarded in her movements on the B.C. trip, being careful with her energy. And Elaine said, "But there was no way that she was slacking one step," which, of course, is exactly Jan. And then she just hit a really bad patch and couldn't go to Alberta.

Jan and I did a performance in Burlington before she got really ill again. I remember watching out the window for her to arrive. And she walked into the church, down the aisle, and came right up the steps to the stage. She said to me, "Wanna see my head?" I nodded, and she whipped off her scarf. Her hair was like a baby's, thin and ragged. It looked so vulnerable, more than a bald head would, I remember thinking. I tried to keep my face neutral, you know, not to look shocked or scared. "Ugly, isn't it?" she said, and she put the scarf back on.

Later, we fussed in the washroom with another scarf. She twisted two ribbons together and I tried to pin them properly at the back. She asked how it looked, and I remember looking back at her reflection in that big mirror and saying, "Dramatic." And it was, really, black and yellow winding together and around her forehead.

But it really hit me at the end. We did the regular introductions after the performance. Jan always says, "I'm Jan Livingston, I'm from Orillia, and I'm a woman living with metastatic breast cancer." I must have heard that a hundred times before. And every time before her voice was strong, saying that. Challenging, even. "I'm a woman *living* with metastatic breast cancer," she would say. You know. Emphasis on the living.

But this time her voice was—I don't know—bitter, maybe. Or defensive. Like she was protecting herself. It made me think, don't we all wish we could protect her.

❋

In Calgary, the response of an audience of health professionals to *Handle with Care?* was particularly memorable. After the performance had ended, an oncologist told the packed room that as he was getting ready to leave for Rounds that morning his daughter asked why he was always leaving so early, and why he was away so much of the time.

Recalling that moment, Ross said that this man's response "was his way of getting into talking about the demands of the job. And that seemed to create a kind of emotional space in the audience. And then the next thing I remember was someone who was obviously even more senior, sitting towards the back of the room, posing the question, 'Is this a good place to have cancer?'"

Several heads turned to face him. "Well, yes, I really think it is," one woman said, perhaps another oncologist. "I think we provide an excellent service." A nurse agreed: "I think we offer some of the best supportive care in the country."

"What do you think?" Ross directed the question back to the oncologist who asked it. 'Is this a good place to have cancer?'

"I think it is," he replied. And then, unexpectedly, his voice broke. The room went silent; people were intent, half-turned in their chairs to face him. "I think it is," he said, fighting to speak. "But it's built on the strength of individuals in this room." We could feel the crowd—nurses, physicians, social workers—taking in his recognition of them, witnessing his pain. Nodding, he spoke the truth of it: "We all have a big, big struggle."

"Then the discussion really centered on how demanding it is to try and do this work, and people obviously feeling quite stretched," said Ross. "People were talking about the need for ways for them to deal with the pain of women's experiences with advanced disease, ways that health professionals can sustain hope for themselves 'in the sea of all that pain,' as one woman said. I really think that was one of the most important experiences with an audience. You felt like something had shifted."

Audiences at *Handle with Care?* and *No Big Deal?* play very much the role that most audiences do when they attend formal theater productions. They sit and watch, sometimes laugh, sometimes cry. Afterwards, we have a discussion period. When the formal discussion ends, people often speak with individual cast members. We can see additional possibilities for audience involvement. Postperformance small group discussions might work well for groups of patients in a workshop context, for example.

Given the type of material we present, however, we would not deliberately seek audience participation during the performance itself. We would avoid the type of scenario described by Denzin, in which "the author can even bring the audience into the performance, do a sing-along, hand out a script, give audience members speaking parts, or make a communal performance out of a scholarly text" (Denzin 1997, 123).

Why do we take this restrained approach to audience participation? Especially in the early performances of *Handle with Care?* we often had smallish audiences. Women with metastatic breast cancer were afraid to attend in case their hope might be undermined. They often chose not to risk an engagement that could increase their vulnerability. Often, the day after a performance, we were invited to come back to the same city and perform again. Those who had seen the production were now able to reassure others that it was funny and helpful and, though difficult in moments, essentially safe. A much larger audience would attend the next performance, they promised. In the prostate cancer production, the audience goes entirely quiet during several monologues in which issues about sexuality and incontinence are aired. This is unspeakable stuff, hard for many men to sit through. In these contexts of danger, it would be unconscionable, we believe, to introduce additional risk.

The same principal applies for health professionals. When interviewed about their response to *Handle with Care?* many noted that seeing the drama on stage gave them the possibility of distance that they were denied in their everyday working lives. At work they are right there, seated across the desk from the crying woman who's just found out she has metastatic disease. But as audience members, they can sit back and watch, freed for once from the need to figure things out, to act in the moment. And with that freedom, they reported being able to see more clearly their own impact on patients, to feel more directly the pain of the people with cancer they work with, and of their own situations.

"Presented dramatically, it gets you at a different level," said a nurse. "It's also that you're removed—not removed, exactly, but being in the audience you're not having to think about the next question, the next response, whether the time's up, your next meeting. It really worked. It's amazing how intense it is, presented this way." Health professionals like this woman valued the distance, the chance to watch; it helped them to reflect on their lives and their practice. We wouldn't want to mess with that.

Our approach in *Handle with Care?* and *No Big Deal?* also stands in contrast to improvisational theater. While we see the potential value for more improvisational types of research-based drama, especially in academic settings where the usual forms of knowledge representation are ripe for maximal disruption, this is not our way.

There are two key reasons for this. First, an improvisational approach may make it less likely that groups under study will recognize themselves on stage, which is one possible criterion by which to judge an ethnographic or performance text (Ellis and Flaherty 1992).

When an actor in the *Handle with Care?* project balked at using the terminology that came from an interview transcript with an oncologist, we told him that this is how oncologists talked when we interviewed them. Speaking their own words back to them is one way they know that they have been understood. It may also be part of what keeps them from walking out in the middle of our presentation at hospital Grand Rounds.

Even more critically, improvisation, except in very limited expressions, replaces the value of a negotiated collective understanding with that of individual expression. The scripts of *Handle with Care?* and *No Big Deal?* emerged from intense and prolonged negotiations across perspectives and across individuals. By the time we agreed on the final script, we were ready to treat our productions, complete with evocative and symbolic scenes, *as if* they were "truth." This was not the revealed truth of a realist tale (Van Maanen 1988), but rather an agreed-upon construction that had been forged through enormous effort and lengthy conversation, privileging the experiences of people with cancer.

Those of us involved with the projects were clear with each other that no individual associated with the productions had the right to mess with these multiply-influenced constructions without reengaging in broader consultation. We agreed to respect the work that had already gone into creating the productions. Actors were expected (although we did not always succeed in these efforts) to speak the exact words in our scripts, using tones and bodily gestures and postures that had been carefully chosen and practiced. Before each new performance, we went over it all again, reminding ourselves, reminding our bodies, of our commitment to getting it "right."

This is not to suggest that we think we have found, or are presenting through our drama, the ultimate truths about cancer, and that no other representations would have value. We are just concerned about being as faithful as possible to our own negotiated version of truth, with its foregrounding of the voices of ill people in our studies. When it comes to performance, then, we abandon our previous commitment to messiness. We seek a performance that is, as much as possible, deliberately fixed in a shape that we have predetermined.

That, of course, is the theory. That is our thoughtful rationale, our crafted commitment to the integrity of the script. And then there was Ross, in Barrie, in the middle of a rehearsal, the week before the first troupe left on the national tour. He was standing at the back of the stage waiting for his turn to speak. He wasn't listening particularly closely. He had rehearsed the show endless times before, and could tell from the rise and fall and pauses of the other voices where they were in the script. And then he heard it: "Research proves that chemo brain is a legitimate problem!" It was Jan, and the line she was saying was an entirely new one.

After the rehearsal, Ross caught up with Jan and asked about the line. Jan explained where she had drawn it from, and said she had checked it out with Vrenia. "I'm kind of uncomfortable with it," Ross said. "It's so—definite." They agreed to drop the line for that evening's performance.

Later, Ross talked with Christina about his experience of this change, and others. "For me it was part of a general kind of 'unraveling' that happened as time went on. Unraveling of the integrity of the script, of the agreements we had made about how it would be performed. None of the changes were horrific in themselves. But I thought, 'We have a script, it's a copyrighted script, we all went to great pains to create this script, why are these things happening?' In a way, I felt it was a violation of the process. And then it's partly my own thing"—he puts on a deep mock-authority voice—"and why don't I know about it?"

Modifications to the script signified two things to Ross. "On the one hand, it made me crazy, like this shouldn't be happening. But I mean the other piece was, people have a sense of ownership of this that's really very positive. It's like they want it to be the best possible. It's part of them, like a finger: if it requires clipping a nail, well, they clip the nail. They don't have to consult anyone to clip the nail. It's their lines, that kind of thing. So I understood it in a way. And valued it even, in a way." He chuckled. "In a little way."

As Ross tells it, the script "unraveled" at another point: a line in the "Hierarchy of Hope" that read, "I hope I live long enough to see this government booted out of office."

"Prior to the national tour, everyone had gone to refresher rehearsals with Vrenia, and I hadn't been part of that," Ross said. "And one of the things she said was, you can do that line here but you can't do it there. You can't do it in British Columbia or Manitoba because they're NDP[2] governments, this sort of thing. And so"—he laughed—"In Barrie, I said, 'It's there in the script and we're going to say it! And Jan, when you go to Manitoba, put it back in the script! It doesn't matter what government it is.' And again, the line is not really the point so much as the fact that it wasn't something that we'd agreed on. So, anyway, they went to Manitoba and the cast revolted. They wouldn't say it. The cast decided that it was offensive to say a line like that in someone else's province. Like, people from Ontario coming in and casting aspersions on another government. So they came back, and I said,"—he makes his voice insistent—"'It doesn't matter! It's in the script!' And I think from then on it got said."

The postperformance discussions were yet another site of departures from agreed-upon protocols. Audience members often asked for advice from us. Early on, we held to the party line: we were not there to give direction. Our aim was to present the issues that came forward in the research.

Later, especially as the national tour progressed, a few people began offering their opinions, suggesting particular paths of action. "That really grew over time, people's desire to give advice," Ross said. "Earlier on you could sort of convince them that they weren't there to be spokespersons. Later it was much harder."

The discussions that followed each performance of *Handle with Care?* were facilitated by one of the cast or a member of the research team. Ten different people took on the role at various times, with health professionals among us usually facilitating discussions in hospitals and Mary Sue or Jan handling community settings.

The facilitator would take comments and questions from the audience, often addressing them him/herself or asking a specific person on stage to answer. Ross and Chris would often answer questions about the research. Mary Sue and Jan would respond to women with breast cancer who commented on their own illness experiences.

The format was one that audiences were used to: comments made, questions asked, responses from the stage. The structure of the discussion carried an implicit assumption that numerous people would have a chance to speak, and thus that the amount of time/space any single person took up was limited. While this was, in part, a constraint, the discussion protocol was intended to help people feel able to make comments about their experiences without having to worry that they would be encouraged to make a public display of feeling. If they did display feeling, they could be reasonably sure that they would not be singled out for an intervention or asked to go into it in more depth. Individuals who were in distress after the performance generally knew where to go for help if they wanted it. They could contact members of the local breast cancer self-help group hosting the evening; they could arrange to see a counselor.

There were also opportunities to talk with other people immediately after the formal discussion. Host organizations usually served refreshments, and people were encouraged to stay and visit. Cast members made a point of mingling with the audience before we started taking down the stage set, providing more private opportunities for interaction. Most intimate exchanges occurred during this postperformance time. Audience members spoke with the cast and one another, asking questions, sharing details of their lives.

While the formal facilitated discussion didn't meet everyone's needs or desires, it seemed better than moving directly from the performance to informal conversations or, even worse, to disbanding immediately. It served as an intermediate zone, helping people bridge between the drama and ordinary discourse.

During the facilitated discussion (and after), audience members often commented on how a particular scene in the drama resonated for them. Many shared stories of their own illness or health care system experiences. And, quite commonly, someone wanted advice: What to do for an ill friend who won't talk about her disease? How to best provide information to patients? How to decide when to stop medical treatment?

Ross was adamant that we not try and answer these questions, that we not exploit the power of our staged performance to set ourselves up as experts. He argued that to become advice-givers would undermine the messages of the drama—that there are many differences among people that formulaic answers are inadequate, even harmful.

As a facilitation strategy, quelling advice-giving had its benefits in keeping us from overextending ourselves. But sometimes it felt unsatisfactory, and this may have contributed to the "unraveling" over time of our commitment to avoid certain kinds of responses to the audience. And as Chris later pointed out, our collective attempt to keep our opinions to ourselves may sometimes have had the unintended affect of making us appear, or even feel, unsympathetic.

Researcher Rant: August 2000: Christina

For me, those postperformance discussions got awkwarder and awkwarder. I couldn't seem to figure out who I "was" in them, who I responded *as*.

Once we were relatively comfortable performing, doing a show would leave us absolutely high. The energy between us rang with achievement. I remember being kind of astonished, after one performance, to see someone in the audience crying. "Oh, yeah," I thought, "This is about hard stuff." And I remember trying to reorganize myself to put that sense of accomplishment aside.

When someone in the audience asked what it was like for those of us who didn't have cancer to be part of *Handle with Care?* I was stumped. Part of me thought, "It's an absolute blast. It's a hoot, a delight. We have a fabulous time." Another voice in my head said, "It's the most fascinating thing: there were all these transcripts, and somehow we're representing them; you've responded, and to what? Is it the words, the images, what is it about drama? The link back to the research—is it there, how does it work, what is its nature?" And then, "It's terribly hard. I have such sadness in it sometimes." And of course, by the time I'd even entered this three-way talk with myself the question would be gone.

This ambivalence about who I was during those discussions was especially activated whenever someone in the audience was acutely upset after the show. I remember a woman telling us, immediately after we had taken our seats on the stage, that her mother had died of metastatic disease when she was seventeen. The drama had spoken to her—screamed at her, perhaps—of all the things she hadn't known: all the ways her mother suffered, all the ways her mother must have felt alone, all the ways she—the daughter—might have contributed to her mother's pain. Her grief was absolute, spilling out into the room of a hundred or so people.

I don't remember how Ross responded; I think one of us said that it hadn't been our intention to make people feel guilty. I know I heard Jan say, immediately, "Your mother knew you were seventeen. Your mother knew you didn't know."

I'm not certain the woman heard Jan's words. And I don't know if it was advice Jan was giving, exactly. But it certainly wasn't a researcher's response, or an actor's. It was a mother, with metastatic breast cancer, speaking to a daughter. Speaking personally. And that's what I wanted for this woman.

When I gave Ross an earlier version of this "Rant," he wrote a lengthy response. He thought I was advocating for an intervention with this woman, and with others, that would "make things better." It's a reasonable assumption: there's no doubt that I have more than my share of "make everything okay" genes in this world. But making it okay, or even better, wasn't my only concern. Again, it was about who we "were" when we responded.

I eventually realized that there was something about the injunction not to give advice that seemed to me to be a prohibition against speaking personally, against saying "I." Since then, in long emails back and forth with Ross, I've come around to thinking that there were circumstances in which it made sense to respond "as" a researcher, and some where it would be okay to answer "as" an actor and participant in creating the drama. But mostly, I wish I had been more alert to the moments when I might have responded more personally, as some kind of witness, someone "in this" with a person in the audience, someone struggling too.

*

CHAPTER TEN
FINAL CURTAIN

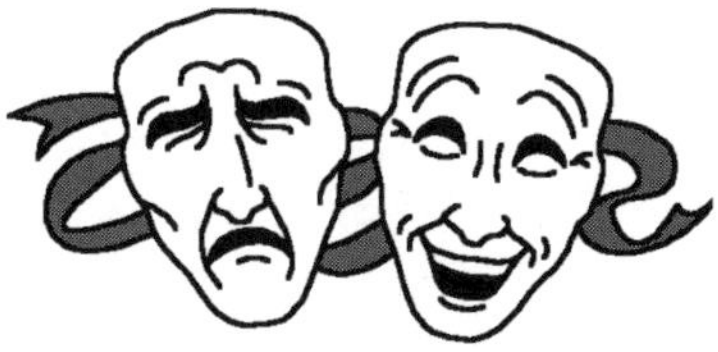

Memorybank Drama: June 2000: Ross

At the reception after our performance at the conference in Vancouver, we behave like actors, by which I mean that we make a beeline for food and drink and keep going back for more. As always, Vrenia is delighted when we take up this starving artist attitude in earnest.

We are high from the performance, and from the standing ovation from the large group of my peers, "psychosocial oncology" professionals. People approach us, tell us how much they enjoyed the show, how wonderful we are. Elaine and Jan confide to us that they've been riding the hotel elevators, greeting adoring fans getting on and off, letting the enthusiasm spill all over them.

I am trying to work my way to the other side of the room where the wine bar is, but there are too many people around me who want to talk about *Handle with Care?* Finally, I manage to extricate myself. I am almost at the bar when I come across Vrenia, deep in animated conversation. She turns to me, eyes aglitter, and introduces me to the woman she's speaking with, a staff member at the Y-Me breast cancer organization in the States.

"Ross, we were just talking about the next Y-Me conference. It's going to be in Chicago next summer and they'd love to have us come. I know you want to be done by then, but I told them we could make an exception. Right?"

I groan. "Vrenia, I'm not going to agree to that. The project is going to be over in a couple of months." She scrunches up her face. "Yeah, but this is such an opportunity!" Not for the first time, I feel like the Grinch who stole Christmas. "That may be, but I don't want anything to do with it. If another group wants to take this on, that's fine, but I'm finished in June."

Having effectively squelched their conversation, I turn away, moving—with more urgency now—towards the wine.

I'd first realized how difficult ending was going to be at a meeting with the entire cast, when I had tried to talk about the project's completion. People spoke about what a shame it would be to end, about how much the drama had come to mean to them, about the good that was being done in the world through our performances. Nobody was willing to discuss a specific end date and I was hard pressed to gain acknowledgment that the project would have to end at all. I was thrown into disarray.

It was my job to raise the money and arrange for performances, so for practical reasons I needed a timeline. I would also, eventually, need to pull back and make room for other projects.

But beyond my own practical issues lay a whole slew of other concerns. Did I have an obligation as a researcher, and as the initiator of this work, to ensure that it had the biggest impact possible? How much return should the participants in the project have a right to expect on their investment of time and life energy? What impact would stopping performances have on Jan and Mary Sue? Several cast members voiced their conviction that *Handle with Care?* was somehow keeping the two women alive. How could we possibly stop?

As I thought about these issues over time, I became convinced of the importance of setting a date for the project to end. Although theoretically one option might have been for me to just drop out, and let things carry on without me, from a practical perspective that would have involved taking the structure of the project apart and setting it up differently under someone else's leadership. The prospect of such a transition seemed daunting.

I also thought that others in the group were, without saying so, looking to me to force the issue of ending. It had been my role to bring this project into being, so it must be my responsibility to initiate its ending. I imagined that people would eventually be thankful for my push to end things. A clean ending would allow them a fresh place to consider possible future participation should there later be a move to reinitiate the project under new terms.

I also felt that to hang on too tightly, too long to the project would only get us into trouble. Some of the actors would get tired, some would drop out, the vitality of the acting would start to wane, the money would run out. There were signs that all of this was already underway. I wanted to be able to embrace the ending, to celebrate our achievements while we were still all enthralled with the project. I didn't want to go through an extended limping towards a reluctant ending.

My conviction that we needed to draw the curtain on the drama was also about death. In the beginning, we had imagined that Death might be a character in the drama, always somewhere on stage, watching and waiting. Although we ended up deciding not to include Death as a character, for me he was still there with us during performances, inching his way towards center stage, his breath growing hotter on the back of my neck. I didn't want to pretend he wasn't there; that he wouldn't eventually take over the stage, that he wouldn't end our project on his terms if we didn't act first.

Finally I decided: my involvement would end in June 2000, three and a half years after the project began and fifteen months after its originally scheduled conclusion. Vrenia and I worked out a set of conditions under which a subgroup of the actors could continue with the show after that date if they so chose. These same conditions would apply to any other theater troupes that might want to mount *Handle with Care?*

I booked the location for a wrap-up party and let everyone know about it. Ending became official. And I promised myself to stay firm about the decision.

In the final analysis, nobody from the *Handle with Care?* troupe coordinated an effort to keep the project alive after its formal conclusion. But people talked a lot about it, and they kept looking to me to change my mind or make exceptions.

In Red Deer, Patricia said jokingly, "Never mind him. He's moved on to more important things with his prostate cancer show. He's abandoned us." Coming back from Victoria, Vrenia and Jan hatched a plan to rewrite the script as a one-woman show for Jan to perform. It would have a totally new look. Rap music would be involved. Cast members started telling me about how various other people in the troupe were struggling with the possibility of ending. At our gala preview of *No Big Deal?* one of the troupe almost undermined a future gig for the prostate cancer show by suggesting to the conference organizer that we instead revive *Handle with Care?* for one special performance. And then, on the night of the final performance of *Handle with Care?* when I was putting away the props for what would be my last time, Vrenia came rushing onto the stage full of ideas about how we could keep the show going.

But by then I felt finished. I had come to feel that the time for ending had arrived.

✻

The final three performances of *Handle with Care?* appeared on the stage of the Robert Gill Theatre in Toronto on June 13, 14, and 15,

2000. Jan and Christina talked about those last shows about a month after they were over.

"I am so resentful that everything was colored by my illness," Jan said. Her brother-in-law had driven her from Orillia to Toronto. "I was feeling shaky all the way down. And when I got to the stairs of the Robert Gill, I thought: 'I've made it.' I almost couldn't believe I was there."

Jan walked slowly from the front steps into the foyer outside the theater. Claudette was there to greet her. Claudette plays the same role Jan does, and had come to the theater ready to perform if Jan didn't feel well enough.

"I was so glad to see Claudette," said Jan. "It meant if I couldn't do it, she was there. It took the pressure off. At the same time, it put some pressure on: 'Damn it, I'm going to do it. I'm going to perform.'"

And perform she did. Dave was among the troupe that worked with Jan the next evening. It was his final show.

"It was very emotional to go through my last performance with Jan," he said. "I wanted it to be so right. I didn't want to goof up—I didn't want to blow any lines, I didn't want to blow any cues, I just wanted to be there for her. And she was, you could just—there was an aura around her that said, 'I'm not feeling strong.' And I thought, okay."

"That night," said Dave, "the cast really came together. You could feel everyone getting the understanding as we went through the rehearsal that we really truly did have to handle this performance with care. This is when we really had to gentle our way through it because it was important to us, to Jan, that we make this cradle of safety for her so that she could be there and perform. And once we were up there and we started, it was really great."

The third night—the very last performance—"Vrenia kind of stirred it up before we went on," Ross remembers. "She said, 'This is the last performance, go for it. Take liberties you haven't taken before,' is basically what she said. Although she would deny it was said quite like that."

In one scene in the drama, the A character, exasperated by her family's demands, thrusts a pile of paper at her husband, the E character, often played by Ross. Each person who took part in this scene had rehearsed it carefully, coordinating the movements so that E could clutch the papers to his chest and move them quickly to the back of the stage.

But a few months prior, just before the national tour had started, one of the women who played A had begun throwing the papers in the air rather than at E directly. Three times the papers had gone all over the stage, and once the performance had to be interrupted so that everyone could gather them up.

Ross had been determined to put an end to this way of doing things. "Vrenia and I ganged up on her—or rather I got Vrenia to help me gang up on her—to convince her not to throw them. We really were putting the screws to her. But it was sort of like she had decided that this was the correct—this was full expression of that moment for her, and it really didn't matter what anybody else said about it."

Christina is listening intently; she didn't see the final performance.

"And so, on the last night," Ross continues, "more than any time in history, she just went straight up in the air with the papers."

"No!" Christina gasps.

"Yeah," he says, and then his voice shifts, becomes intense, incredulous: "And I caught them all on the way down."

"You're kidding."

He laughs. "It was like some superhuman feat. There was a kind of response from the audience, I don't know, they might have clapped. And you know that scene where the doctor is saying 'blah blah blah'? Before the show, Vrenia said to me, 'Take that scene as long as you want. Draw pictures on the desk.' So I did. And in other places as well. But it was a bit scary. Would we put it over the top in a way that would undermine the script—would it become a kind of showcase? It was very unnerving in a certain kind of way while at the same time quite delicious and energizing."

"What would have happened, if it did go over the edge?" Christina asks.

"It wouldn't have been a disaster I guess," Ross replies. "But I didn't want it to be an in-joke. That's what I worried about. There are the people who know all about it, and there are some people out there who've never seen this before. And it hurts, right? So I was like . . . I didn't want it to become about us, doing our last performance. I still wanted it to be about the audience. But the entire evening was sort of a razor's edge thing. Vrenia was pushing Mary Sue to do Magda twice as big as she'd done it before."

And Mary Sue did, drawing the scene out, reveling in it, her long arms waving the black boa through the air.

"Ta Dah! I'm Invisible!" from the *Handle with Care?* Script

Ladies and gentlemen, step right up and see Magda, the magician. With a few magic words, I can make things disappear. I can even make myself disappear. Just a simple magic formula—easier than Abracadabra.

Well, I don't exactly disappear. After I utter those magic words, a cloud will descend on you and you will no longer see me.

You don't believe me?

Wait and see. I've done it before, with friends and family and it's surefire, no-fail.

And what is this magic formula, you ask?

Ready!—here goes!

But first, take a good look at me and remember what I look likc.

And now—Ta Dah! (DRUM ROLL) the FIVE MAGIC WORDS:

I Have Metastatic Breast Cancer. (E STRIKES BELL ONCE)

So, do you still see me or has the cloud done its work?

Some of you do? How unusual! The same me you saw before? Without the usual masks? The mask of the doomed woman, the mask of the victim, the mask of the invalid, the mask of the heroine, the fighter!

Where's the real me? The one who loves chocolate fudge and Robert Redford movies? Who wants to play bridge, talk about your son's wedding, hold my niece's new baby? The one who wants to share your joys and sorrows as much as I ever did?

I wish I had a magic formula to make that woman come back, from under the cloud, from behind the masks. If any of you know that one, please tell me.

"I didn't get Magda right from the beginning," Mary Sue confessed a few weeks after that final performance. "I didn't really get what she was saying, because I think I was worried about remembering the words, and Vrenia was teaching me what to do. I wasn't really listening to Magda.

"I couldn't believe when Vrenia kept saying, 'make it bigger.' I'd think, 'What are you talking about?' And I'd try, and think I was over the top, but probably not until the last night, and probably it could have been bigger than that. Had Vrenia tried to get that out of me in the beginning I would have felt so intimidated I guess, and foolish. But each time she got a little bit bigger and Vrenia would explain a little bit more, because she could see what it was, she could see all of the things that I couldn't.

"I always loved doing Magda, and most recently even more, because the audience is very silent. They're trying to get it, they're trying to understand who she is and what she's trying to say. It's a wonderful connection."

Mary Sue pauses, reflecting on the scene.

"I think Magda is saying, 'I'm the same person I was before, please see that.' And that's what I wanted people to hear and see when I played her. But it took me a while to get it."

Mary Sue's son Trevor brought a friend of his, Nicole, to the final *Handle with Care?* performance. "Nicole wrote me a really lovely note afterwards," Mary Sue said. "And at the bottom of it she wrote, 'I do see you.' And I thought—she doesn't know me very well, I've only met her a few times—but she really got it. It was really neat."

From Elaine

I'm probably not fully acknowledging the finality of the last shows because to me it could never be over. That is nothing to do with hanging on—it's just that there's too much in it for me to say it's over. It's not over for me.

From Mary Sue

I'm glad we got the opportunity to get to know people, because it made this a unique experience. I don't know whether you need to do that in another project, but it made this wonderful, because that happened.

From Patricia

It was such wonderful laughter that we had. Tears as well, but I really think we had more laughter than tears.

I can't believe we're not going to do it again. I just can't believe it.

From Jan

I think that for whatever reasons, fate met in this moment in my life. My theater background and my educational background, and to be having metastatic cancer, all sort of met on this plane. It's like it was meant to be somehow.

From Ann

Being engaged in this kind of project in a way transforms the suffering. It's so easy to romanticize and say that it's going to change things. That's maybe wishful thinking. But it's as if suffering becomes raw material for something else as opposed to being an end place where one winds up.

From Vrenia

The story underneath the story is about a journey we took to come together as a real group, all taking ownership in the project with nobody standing on the outside. People presented themselves generously, opened the shutters. It was profoundly painful and it was joyful in equal measure.

Researcher Rant: August 2000: Christina

At the outset of *Handle with Care?* our roles were undefined, the nature and extent of our involvement in this project uncharted. Uncertainty threaded through our engagement with the subject and with one another. No one person had all of the pieces. Professionals in one arena were lay people in the other. The researchers knew nothing of creating a drama. Most of the members of Act II Studio came relatively new to both drama and research; for many, metastatic was a new word.

Over the course of the project, each person "took on" more and more pieces. We learned that Patricia, and other women from Act II Studio, had experienced a breast cancer diagnosis, and one woman's husband was undergoing chemotherapy. Ross and Christina became actors. Jan assumed significant stage management responsibilities and wrote key dramatic scenes. By the time a script was generated, Vrenia could quote from and identify the oncologist transcripts by number. Friendships formed. At this point, the way we categorize ourselves—actors, researchers, women with the disease—seems stark and less than truthful.

In reflecting on how the *Handle with Care?* troupe had come together, Jan expressed both appreciation and a kind of surprise: "I was really impressed that the actors stayed with it. Because I think the potential to be frightened off was huge. . . . None of them have been unscathed by cancer, you know."

Handle with Care? affirmed in multiple ways the virtues of hanging in, of getting and staying involved. As a research and a theatrical undertaking—and, indeed, as a human adventure—the project turned on the dangerous possibilities of relationships, on the multiple and sometimes contrary cultural meanings of "closeness."

Both linguistically and culturally, "closeness" contains risk, danger, and vulnerability: a close call, too close for comfort, close to the bone. "Distance" contains meanings around both professionalism and safety. These meanings also emerge in discussions about ethical research practice. Miles and Huberman (1994) organize theoretical frameworks around fieldwork ethics along a kind of continuum, with "avoidance of harm" congruent with a utilitarian framework and "avoidance of detachment" at the other end.

In *Handle with Care?* our attention to the experience of living with metastatic breast cancer was "close," was analytically, imaginatively, and personally engaged. We were—and are—

attached. Elaine said it best: the title of the drama, she said, "has two dimensions. *Handle with Care?* can be standoffish. But I think the way we look at it is, *Handle with Caring*. That isn't as good as a title, but it is *Handle with Caring*. Because if we look at it from its fragile sense, we'll stand too far back."

Handle with Care? then, in both its title and our experiences in it, contains meanings which might have kept us at a distance—frightened us off, or rendered us unhelpfully tentative. If we had looked at it, or at one another, as (only) fragile or dangerous, we may well have stood too far back. As it was, we were close enough to understand, and close enough to act.

Researcher Rant: August 2000: Ross

Lots of people have told us they were afraid to come to a performance about the scary topic of metastatic breast cancer. But those who attended *Handle with Care?* left feeling more hopeful than they'd expected; not hoping for miracle cures, but for the possibility of living fully, the possibility of humor, of connection, and of grace, in the face of enormous difficulties and limited time.

What generates hope? A while back, I received a call for abstracts for a conference with hope and illness as its major themes. I wanted to present something about *Handle with Care?* As I reflected on the transcripts from our focus groups of women with metastatic breast cancer, I became convinced that hope does not just reside in content. Hope throws us into the middle of such a thorny topic. It pushes us to make a difference. Hope is in motion. It bounds across the stage. It rolls around in suffering and makes light of it at the same time. Hope is much more than a topic; it lives in creative engagement.

*

EPILOGUE

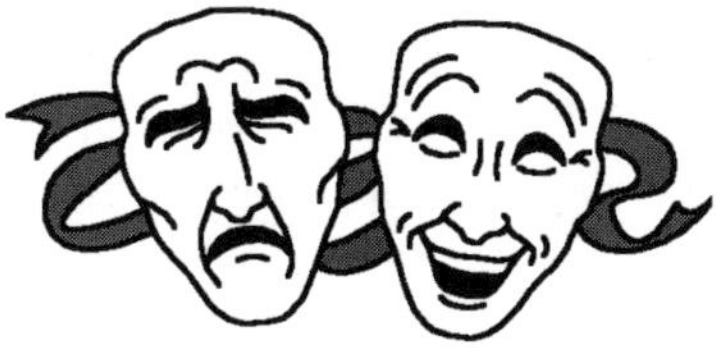

Christina, Just Talking: September 2000

In July, between long stretches at the computer shifting and sorting chapter 7, Ann and I drove to Orillia to see Jan. I took my tape recorder, hoping that we could have a conversation about the national tour and the final *Handle with Care?* performances. I had talked with Jan the night before to make sure she was still up for a visit. She sounded pleased we were coming, and a bit relieved; she was still feeling ill and depleted (her physicians blamed a stubborn inner ear infection), and Ann and I could be "on duty" to help out if needed.

Much about seeing her that day was a gift: Jan has a knack for storytelling, and a generous honesty about herself, and both shone as we talked. Or, perhaps it's more true to say they shone through—through pain, and through the utter tiredness of being ill for so long—often flickering, sometimes bright.

Transcribing the tape the next day and trying to figure out how to knit what Jan had said into the final chapters, I could feel the energy of my writing ebbing.

Yes, the illness has been present in everything we've done. And that bubbling fear, and that yearning for it to all go away, has intruded before. But it's different now. What we did together was so buoyant; it carried us along, and it has carried me in this writing. I don't feel carried anymore.

Barely a week after we were at her home, Jan ended up back in the hospital. Metastases had appeared in bones in her leg and shoulder. She had surgery to stabilize her leg and was then flown to Sudbury for more radiation. She was home, briefly, and then back in the hospital at the end of August, with fractures.

Email from Christina, August 28, 2000

Hi, everyone.

Four of us—Ann, Falia (who I work with at Willow, for those of you who don't know her), me and Elaine (one of the Handle with Care? *troupe, for the rest), went to Orillia yesterday to see Jan. She was surprised to see us: our plan had been to go up today, but her sister Judy called to say Jan might leave again for Sudbury, so we gathered ourselves together and drove up Sunday.*

We walked into her room, and (so that she wouldn't have to repeat herself), we all stood for a few moments while Jan gave us the latest medical updates. Then she said, "I'm scared and I'm angry and life pretty much sucks right now." And we all pretty much agreed with her.

Then Ann and Elaine and I went out, and Falia spent a few moments with her; then Falia left, and Ann went in; then Elaine, and then me; we left a bit of time in between so she could rest. Ann said she stroked Jan's legs and massaged her feet.

I told Jan about all the phone calls and email messages winding back and forth about her and she smiled at this. She said she had received a bunch of cards with hearts on them from the Handle with Care? *crew. It clearly means lots to her that we're all thinking about her, and talking with one another.*

When her mother arrived I left, and Jan said, "give my love to everyone."

So love, to all, from Jan.
xoxo
Chris

Email from Christina, August 28, 2000

Ross:

Ann told me that she and Jan had talked about Handle with Care? *and Jan said she didn't regret one moment of it. She said, "I've made my mark."*

xoxo
Chris

Early in October, one of the *Handle with Care?* cast members, Barbara Haber, hosted a gathering. It was a kind of reunion, almost two years to the day since our very first performance in Kingston.

It was clear, then, that Jan was dying. When Ross and Christina had visited the week before, she was in and out of consciousness, and very weak.

The day of the party, Christina called Elaine, and then Mary Sue, and then Ross, and we fretted and puzzled together over how we might properly "recognize" Jan—celebrate her, and acknowledge her suffering—while not making the entire event about her, or about mourning. She had not died, after all; this was not a memorial, and it was not a gathering we had orchestrated.

We decided to bring along a video of the performance in Orillia, with Jan absolutely radiant, floating on the applause of hundreds of people in the Opera House theater, and a few readings we each liked. We mapped out a tentative plan for beginning a conversation about Jan.

When we got there, it was harder. Everyone chatted, caught up, and had good food. Jan was absent.

As the evening wore on, we sat in our separate parts of the room, scrambling in our heads to figure it out. Were people less connected to Jan than we'd thought? Had they all had their own conversations, elsewhere, and settled their sadness? Were they waiting for one of us to speak?

At one point, someone mentioned Vrenia and Sandy's "high tea" adventure at the Empress Hotel in Victoria. "Jan really loved that you did that," Christina said. The air stilled.

"Yeah, I really miss Jan," someone commented, offhand—and turned to another topic.

Later, in more private conversations as we were clearing up, several people did ask about Jan, and one woman remarked on Christina's effort to "bring Jan into the room." As Mary Sue said afterwards as well, both the composition and the dynamic of the group had changed since we had all traveled together; patterns of attention and intimacy had shifted.

At the same time, of course, it was also pretty clear that we were, once again, in an awkward dance of silence, sliding gracelessly around the most disruptive truths of metastatic breast cancer.

Our laughter and our hope had banished Death, sent her scuttling from the room. Now, she was with us again, sitting on the couch, drinking our wine. And none of us wanted to look at her face.

Email from Mary Sue, October 12, 2000

Hi Christina.

I thought about the gathering at Barbara's all day yesterday. I had the crummy flu so vague thoughts came through between sleeps. Also read some of the Standing Ovation *manuscript which brought back lots of memories—tears and laughter—struggles with Death stalking the room! We did think we had it all figured out.*

I felt a little at odds about the evening. Several times I was just going to speak out but I didn't. And then when the few of us were talking after the party, I thought everyone in the group would have had something to add so I was really sorry that I hadn't blurted out something earlier.

On another note, Patricia came to the public lecture series last night. It was a shame she wasn't able to attend the party. It was great fun to see her—she looks terrific and we had a wonderful hug and a short visit.

Another thought I had [lonely as thoughts are !!]: the dynamics of the group are changing, and have been for quite a while, and that's the way it should be. Life changes and we all move on. Oh boy, so profound.

Love you lots and lots
M.S.

Ross, Just Talking: October 2000

I am thinking a lot about Jan these days. Often, in the evenings, I do some Buddhist chanting for her, using the same drum that we used on the *Handle with Care?* stage. My voice immersed in the ancient tones and rhythms, I focus on the picture we had taken in Florida, Jan beaming in the middle.

I find it is less the particular expression of the chanting that is important, and more what it allows. A way of staying connected with her across distance, holding her in attention. A way of reaching out, sending love.

None of it takes the pain away, but, then, I wasn't expecting to get rid of the pain.

*

Jan died on October 15, 2000.

*

Christina, Just Talking: October 2000

Ever the stage manager, Jan had left instructions about the tone and organization of her funeral. At her request, both Ross and I spoke about *Handle with Care?* her contribution to it, and how much it had meant to her. I was also one of the eight—all women—pallbearers.

Elaine arranged that the *Handle with Care?* troupe would be an honor guard at Jan's funeral. My most loved memory from that day is of walking beside her coffin as it wheeled out of the church, and looking up to see the people who had created and acted in *Handle with Care?* I expected them to be lined up, separate, facing ahead; my image was, I think, military. And yet, there they were—holding hands, stretched out along the sidewalk. Ross. Patricia. Elaine. Mary Sue. Vrenia. Ann. Fran. Claudette. Ruth. Sandra. Sandy. Barbara.

Not an honor guard—an honor chain. A human chain. Everyone linked. Everyone holding on. Everyone handling one another, with care.

NOTES

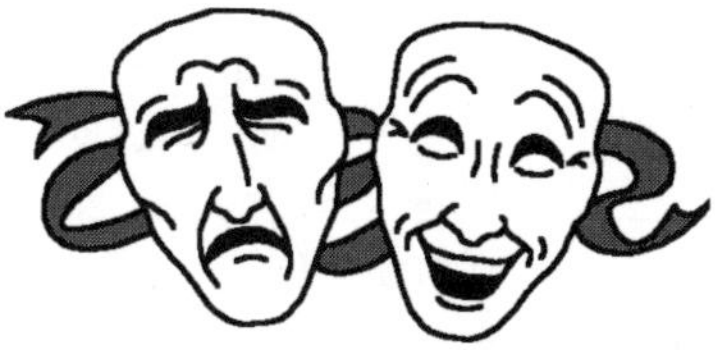

Acknowledgments

1. In each city or town, we usually performed to both health professional and community audiences. We visited several of these communities on more than one occasion.

Chapter 1

1. Act II Studio is a theater school and creative drama center for adults over age fifty at Ryerson Polytechnic University in Toronto.

2. Some examples: Bedford 1999; Canadian Press 1999; Cole 2000; Gee 2000, 31; Gordon 1999; Jarvis 1998; Kearsey 2000, A4; Peters 1999, 54; Senick 2000; Stacey 2000; Zacharjewicz 1999.

3. Produced by Lynda Shorten as part of CBC Radio's "Real Life with Cancer" series, the audio documentary follows Jan Livingston through the day *Handle with Care?* performs in her hometown to a sell-out crowd, interviewing her about her experience with the drama and her life with metastatic disease. More information: http://radio.cbc.ca/programs/thismorning/features/cancer.html.

4. Directed and produced by Laura Sky, the documentary *How Can We Love You? Behind the Scenes with the Play* Handle with Care? weaves excerpts from the drama together with Mary Sue's and Jan's personal stories. The camera follows the cast of *Handle with Care?* across the continent as we tour, rehearse, perform, and spend time with one another. The documentary also captures audience responses to the drama. More information: www.laurasky.org.

Chapter 2

1. Cheeseman directed *Hands Up—For You the War Is Ended* in 1971 and *Fight for Shelton Bar* in 1974

2. Major research-derived productions—related to schizophrenia, substance abuse, and sexual assault—have been mounted by Mienczakowski's team. In the process of developing this work, they have provided detailed articulations of the processes of translating research into theater script and performance (Mienczakowski 1996a; Mienczakowski 1999) and have also offered cogent theoretical arguments that create a foundation of relevance for research-based theater (Mienczakowski 1996b; Mienczakowski 1997). Mienczakowski suggests, for instance, that drama has advantages over purely textual reports in terms of validity (i.e., remaining true to qualitative research data and ultimately to lived reality). In part, this can be because it sustains connections to bodies, emotions, and the full range of sensory experience that was present in the original data-gathering situation. Audiences, often comprised of members of groups under study, further validate research-based drama through provision of post-performance feedback, potentially affecting the shape of future presentations (Mienczakowski 1996a).

3. Denzin excuses Mienczakowski from this criticism; Mienczakowski's work, despite its commitment to verisimilitude, is explicitly engaged in cultural critique.

Chapter 9

1. According to the QiGong Research Society (www.qigongresearchsociety.com), Qi is the vital energy or the universal essence that flows throughout the human body and all living things. The Oxford Dictionary describes Qi as "the physical life force postulated by certain Chinese philosophers to flow through the body."

2. New Democratic Party, Canada's political left.

REFERENCES

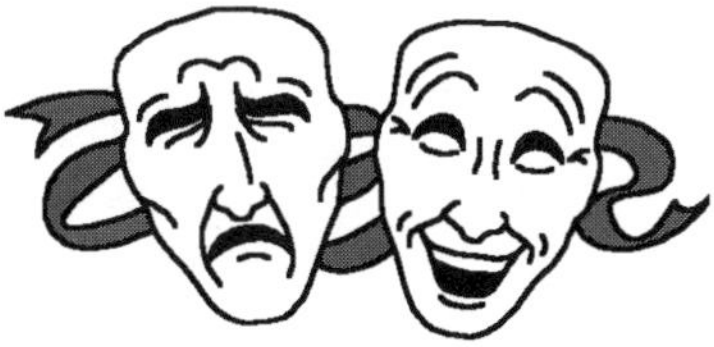

Becker, H. S., M. M. McCall, and L. V. Morris. 1989. "Theatres and communities: Three scenes." *Social Problems* 36:93–116.

Bedford, Frances. 1999. "Acting and healing combine at Sunnybrook." *The North Toronto Post*. Toronto, Ontario.

Behar, R. 1996. *The vulnerable observer*. Boston: Beacon Press.

Bologh, R. 1981. "Grounding the alienation of self and body: A critical, phenomenological analysis of the patient in western medicine." *Sociology of Health and Illness* 3:188–206.

Brady, S. 1999. "Looking for Lecoq: A master's legacy lives on." Theatre Communications Group.

Canadian Press. 1999. "Breast cancer patients seek respect on stage." *The Toronto Star*. Toronto, Ontario.

Church, K. 1995. *Forbidden narratives*. Amsterdam: Gordon & Breach.

Cole, Sally. 2000. "Cancer patients tell story through *Handle with Care?*" *The Guardian*. Charlottetown, Prince Edward Island.

Collins, P. H. 1990. *Black feminist thought: Knowledge, consciousness, and the politics of empowerment*. Boston: Unwin, Hyman.

Conquergood, D. 1991. "Rethinking ethnography: Towards a critical cultural politics." *Communications monographs* 58:170–94.

———. 1992. "Ethnography, rhetoric, and performance." *Quarterly journal of speech* 78:80–97.

Denzin, N. 1997. *Interpretive ethnography*. Thousand Oaks, Calif.: Sage.

Ellis, C. 1991. "Emotional sociology." *Studies in symbolic interaction* 12:123–45.

Ellis, C., and L. Berger. 2002. "Their story/my story/our story: Including the researcher's experience in interview research." In *The handbook of interview research: Context and method*, edited by J. Gubrium and J. Holstein. Thousand Oaks, Calif.: Sage.

Ellis, C., and A. P. Bochner. 1992. "Telling and performing personal stories: The constraints of choice in abortion." In *Investigating subjectivity: Research on lived experience*, edited by C. Ellis and M. Flaherty. Newbury Park, Calif.: Sage.

Ellis, C., and M.G. Flaherty. 1992. "An agenda for the interpretation of lived experience." In *Investigating subjectivity: Research on lived experience*, edited by C. Ellis and M. G. Flaherty. Newbury Park, Calif.: Sage.

Fonow, M. M., and J. Cook. 1991. "Back to the future: A look at the second wave of feminist epistemology and methodology." In *Beyond methodology: Feminist scholarship as lived research*, edited by M. M. Fonow and J. Cook. Bloomington: Indiana University Press.

Gastaldo, D. 1997. "Is health education good for you? Rethinking health education through the concept of biopower." In *Foucault, health, and medicine*, edited by A. Peterson and R. Bunton. London: Routledge.

Gee, Skana. 2000. "Play brings breast cancer research to life." *The Daily News*. Halifax, Nova Scotia.

Gingrich-Philbrook, C. 1998. "What I 'know' about the story (for those about to tell personal narrative on stage)." In *The future of performance studies: Visions and revisions*, edited by S. J. Dailey. Annandale: National Communication Association.

Goffman, E. 1963. *Stigma: Notes on the management of spoiled identity*. Englewood Cliffs, N.Y.: Prentice Hall.

Gordon, Kennedy. 1999. "Reality on stage." *The Sudbury Star*. Sudbury, Ontario.

Gray, R. 2000. "Graduate school never prepared me for this: Reflections on the challenges of research-based theatre." *Reflective practice* 1:377–90.

Gray, R., M. Fitch, C. Phillips, M. Labrecque, and K. Fergus. 2000. "Managing the impact of illness: The experiences of men with prostate cancer and their spouses." *Journal of health psychology* 5:525–42.

Gray, R., M. Greenberg, M. Fitch, C. Sawka, A. Hampson, M. Labrecque, and B. Moore. 1998. "Information needs of women with metastatic breast cancer." *Cancer prevention and control* 2:57–62.

Gray, R., V. Ivonoffski, and C. Sinding. (2002). "Making a mess and spreading it around: Articulation of a model for research-based drama." In *Ethnographically Speaking: Autoethnography, literature, and aesthetics*, edited by A. Bochner and C. Ellis. Walnut Creek, Calif.: AltaMira Press.

Gray, R., C. Sinding, and M. Fitch. (2001). "Navigating the social context of metastatic breast cancer: Reflections on a project linking research to drama." *Health* 5: 233–48.

Gray, R., C. Sinding, V. Ivonoffski, M. Fitch, A. Hampson, and M. Greenberg. 2000. "The use of research-based theatre in a project related to metastatic breast cancer." *Health expectations* 3:137–44.

Hall, J. D., J. Leloudis, R. Korstad, M. Murphy, L. A. Jones, and C. B. Daly. 1987. *Like a family: The making of a southern cotton mill world.* Chapel Hill: University of North Carolina Press.

Illich, I. 1976. *Medical nemesis: The expropriation of health.* London: Calder & Boyars.

Ivonoffski, V., and R. Gray. 1998. "Handle with care? Women living with metastatic breast cancer." Unpublished performance script.

———. 1999. "No Big Deal?" Unpublished performance script.

Jackson, M. 1989. *Paths towards a clearing: Radical empiricism and ethnographic inquiry*. Bloomington: Indiana University Press.

Jackson, S. 1993. "Ethnography and the audition: Performance as ideological critique." *Text and Performance Quarterly* 13:21–43.

Jagger, A. 1989. "Love and knowledge: Emotion in feminist epistemology." *Inquiry* 32:151–76.

Jarvis, Anne. 1998. "Cancer study inspires play." *The Windsor Star*. Windsor, Ontario.

Kaufman, M. 2000. "Into the west: An exploration in form." Theatre Communications Group.

Kearsey, Tara. 2000. "Overcoming the silence." *Yellowknifer*. Yellowknife, Northwest Territories.

Laurence, M. 1974. *The diviners.* Toronto: Bantam.

Marcus, G. E. 1994. "What comes (just) after 'post'? The case of ethnography." In *The handbook of qualitative research*, edited by N. K. Denzin and Y. S. Lincoln. Thousand Oaks, Calif.: Sage.

Mathews, H. F., D. R. Lannin, and J. P. Mitchell. 1994. "Coming to terms with advanced breast cancer: Black women's narratives from eastern North Carolina." *Social science and medicine* 38:789–800.

Mayer, M. 1998. *Advanced breast cancer: A guide to living with metastatic disease*. Cambridge: O'Reilly & Associates.

McCall, M. M. 1993. "Not just a farmer and not just a farm wife." Unpublished performance script.

———. 2000. "Performance ethnography: A brief history and some advice." In *The handbook of qualitative research*. Vol. 2, edited by N. K. Denzin and Y. S. Lincoln. Thousand Oaks, Calif.: Sage.

McCall, M. M., and H. S. Becker. 1990. "Performance science." *Social problems* 37:117–32.

Mienczakowski, J. 1996a. "An ethnographic act: The construction of consensual theatre." In *Composing ethnography: Alternative forms of writing*, edited by C. Ellis and A. Bochner. Walnut Creek, Calif.: AltaMira Press.

———. 1996b. "On the road to catharsis: A theoretical framework for change." *Qualitative inquiry* 2:439–62.

———. 1997. "Theatre of change." *Research in drama education* 2:159–72.

———. 1999. "Ethnography in the hands of participants: Tools of dramatic discovery." In *Studies in educational ethnography*. Vol. 2, *Explorations in Methodology*, edited by G. Walford and A. Massey. Oxford: JAI Press.

Mienczakowski, J., and S. Morgan. 1994. "Ethnographic drama research: Combining research, creativity, and performance." In *Synching out loud: A journey into illness*. Vol. 2. Brisbane, Australia: Reprographics, Griffith University.

Miles, M. B., and A. M. Huberman. 1994. "Ethical issues in analysis." In *Qualitative data analysis*. Thousand Oaks, Calif.: Sage.

Mills, C. W. 1959. *The sociological imagination*. New York: Oxford.

Morgan, K. P. 1998. "Contested bodies, contested knowledges: Women, health, and the politics of medicalization." In *The politics of women's health: Exploring agency and autonomy*, edited by S. Sherwin. Philadelphia: Temple University Press.

Narayan, U. 1988. "Working together across difference: Some considerations on emotions and political practice." *Hypatia* 3:31–47.

Paget, D. 1987. "'Verbatim theatre': Oral history and documentary techniques." *New theatre quarterly* 12:317–36.

Paget, M. 1983. "On the work of talk: Studies in misunderstandings." In *The social organization of doctor-patient communication*, edited by S. Fisher and A. Dundas-Todd. Washington, D.C.: Center for Applied Linguistics.

———. 1993. *A complex sorrow: Reflections on cancer and an abbreviated life*, edited by M. L. DeVault. Philadelphia: Temple University Press.

Park-Fuller, L. 2000. "Performing absence: The staged personal narrative as testimony." *Text and performance quarterly* 20:20–42.

Pelias, R. J. 1999. *Writing performance: Poeticizing the researcher's body*. Carbondale: Southern Illinois University Press.

Peters, Diane 1999. "Breast cancer culture." *Chatelaine*, November.

Pollock, D. 1990. "Telling the told: Performing like a family." *Oral history review* 18:1–36.

Richardson, L. 1994. "Writing as a method of inquiry." In *The handbook of qualitative research*, edited by N. K. Denzin and Y. S. Lincoln. Thousand Oaks, Calif.: Sage.

Scheman, N. 1995. "Feminist epistemology." *Metaphilosophy* 26:177–190.

Senick, Dave. 2000. "Touring breast cancer drama helps expose taboo subject." *Times Colonist*. Victoria, British Columbia.

Sherwin, S. 1998. "A relational approach to autonomy in health care." In *The politics of women's health*, edited by S. Sherwin. Philadelphia: Temple University Press.

Sinding, C., R. Gray, M. Fitch, and M. Greenberg. (2002). "Staging breast cancer, rehearsing metastatic disease." *Qualitative health research* 12: 61–73.

Smith, A. D. 1993. *Fires in the mirror: Crown Heights, Brooklyn, and other identities*. Garden City, N.Y.: Anchor.

———. 1994. *Twilight: Los Angeles, 1992*. Garden City, N.Y.: Anchor.

Stacey, Jean Edwards. 2000. "Drama with a message." *The Telegram*. St. John's, Newfoundland.

Stake, R. 1994. "Case studies." In *The handbook of qualitative research*, edited by N. Denzin and Y. Lincoln. Thousand Oaks, Calif.: Sage.

Stucky, N. 1993. "Toward an aesthetics of natural performance." *Text and performance quarterly* 13:168–80.

Trinh, T. M-ha. 1991. *When the moon waxes red: Representation, gender, and cultural politics*. New York: Routledge.

Turner, B. 1992. *Regulating bodies: Essays in medical sociology*. London: Routledge.

Turner, V. 1986. *The anthropology of performance*. New York: PAJ Publications.

Van Maanen, J. 1988. *Tales of the field: On writing ethnography*. Chicago: University of Chicago Press.

Walstrom, N. 1996. "'Mystory' of anorexia nervosa: New discourses for change and recovery." *Cultural studies: A research annual* 1:67–99.

Williams, S. 1987. "Goffman, interactionism, and the management of stigma in everyday life." In *Sociological theory and medical sociology*, edited by G. Scambler. New York: Tavistock.

Zacharjewicz. 1999. "Cancer studies explored in theatrical format." *Espanola/Manitoulin Recorder*. Espanola, Ontario.

ABOUT THE AUTHORS

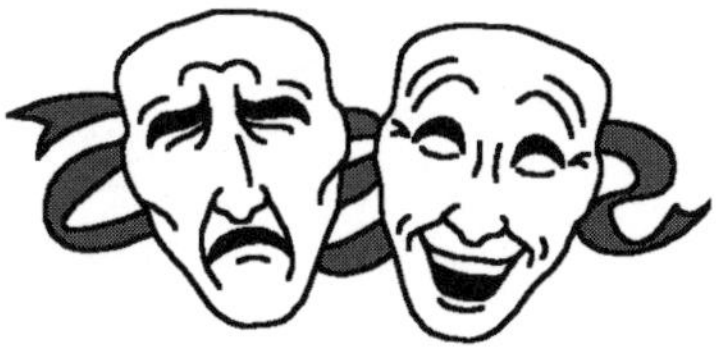

Ross Gray is codirector of the Psychosocial and Behavioural Research Unit, Toronto Sunnybrook Regional Cancer Centre. He is also assistant professor, Department of Public Health Sciences, University of Toronto.

Christina Sinding is a social scientist with the Canadian Breast Cancer Foundation Community Research Initiative. She is currently completing her Ph.D. thesis in the Department of Public Health Sciences, University of Toronto.